The new
reversing s)   restoring
hormone b   ..ce, mental health,
and fertility for good.

Jane Kennedy

PCOS - The New Science of Completely Reversing Symptoms

Jane Kennedy

Published by Jane Kennedy, 2019.

While every precaution has been taken in the preparation of this book, the publisher assumes no responsibility for errors or omissions, or for damages resulting from the use of the information contained herein.

PCOS - THE NEW SCIENCE OF COMPLETELY REVERSING SYMPTOMS

First edition. October 6, 2019.

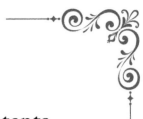

Table of Contents

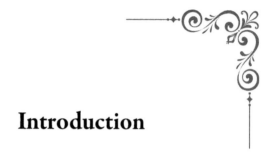

Introduction

A PCOS diagnosis can be frustrating, even devastating news. But it is not as bad as it seems. With knowledge of the condition, those with PCOS can properly arm themselves with effective tools to improve their health, both physical and mental, by educating themselves with the latest information on the subject.

In this book, you will find compiled a source of the latest studies and research on the disease explained in an understandable way, as well as information on improving your own mental health issues you may be having as a result of PCOS, both diagnosed and undiagnosed, such as depression, stress, and guilt.

Women are tired of going to the doctor and hearing the same advice when it comes to PCOS and their fertility! Lose weight. Exercise. Get pregnant. That's what it all seems to amount to.

While losing excess weight is good advice, in fact, it is still probably the best advice for those with PCOS, studies show that it is considerably harder and slower for women with the condition to do so. On top of this, frustration with weight loss can increase stress factors and other mental health issues, making it harder to stay motivated.

This book attempts to take a different approach, which is to take the generic advice commonly heard and pair it with specific, applicable research to create an action plan suitable for your exact needs while remembering to acknowledge emotional issues those afflicted with PCOS face on a sometimes daily basis. **You will not find another book that is focused exclusively on non-diet related methods of treating PCOS**.

And if you do decide to pursue weight loss as well as an avenue for treatment, a diet specifically designed for your needs is suggested and I have intentionally separated this information into a companion piece, "The PCOS Diet," by myself, Jane Kennedy.

Many symptoms, such as facial hair growth, can be *significantly* reduced using insulin and hormone control methods, while others can be reversed and eliminated completely and sometimes permanently.

Arm yourself with the most current available knowledge on polycystic ovarian syndrome, while remembering that this is something that happened to you, not something you did.

Don't waste any more time before beginning to walk the road to freedom from acne, hair loss, and other symptoms that only get worse over time.

If your goal is to increase fertility, you're all too aware that the sooner you begin, the better.

There's no need to wait any longer before reversing the direction that PCOS is taking you and, instead, taking the steps to a calmer, happier life. Let's begin.

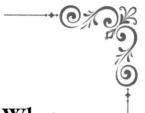

Chapter One: What Is PCOS? A Brief Overview

Polycystic Ovary Syndrome (PCOS) may be a difficult diagnosis, especially since it is not a well-known issue, despite a large number of women suffering from it. Every woman's symptoms manifest themselves differently, and there is not a lot of information available about PCOS.

One goal of this book is to let you know that you are NOT alone. Another goal is to let you know that there is a lot of hope for reducing, and even reversing, some of your symptoms, if not all of them. A third goal is to help you find the resources and information you need to help you and your doctor find the right treatment plan for you.

Consider this shocking statistic shared by Professor Helena Teede, a leading expert on PCOS: "More than 80 percent of women surveyed by the ABC said they felt there was not enough information available about the condition and more than half said they had never heard of PCOS prior to their diagnosis."

The good news is that the international health community has taken notice of this lack of information, and they have taken steps to correct it. Researchers and consortiums, consisting of experts on PCOS, are conducting new studies every year with the aim of identifying the causes and treatments for this syndrome. The ongoing research will help doctors diagnose the syndrome sooner, and help determine the right treatment for you. This is especially important, since each woman's symptoms manifest themselves differently, meaning that each woman will need a specialized treatment plan.

What Is PCOS?

PCOS occurs when women produce higher amounts of male hormones than is normal. The ovaries produce estrogen and progesterone, which are hormones that regulate the menstrual cycle. The ovaries also produce small amounts of androgens, which are male hormones. When ovaries produce too much androgen, this causes PCOS.

The excess androgen produced is usually testosterone. All women need and produce testosterone, just like all males need and produce small amounts of estrogen (even if they do not want to admit it). However, when overproduced, the male hormones start interfering with your body.

You have two main hormones that are responsible for telling your ovaries when to allow one of your eggs to mature and when the egg should be released. This, of course, is ovulation. These two hormones must be working properly for you to ovulate and then, if the egg is not fertilized, for you to menstruate, eliminating your egg from the body. The follicle-stimulating hormone (FSH) causes the ovaries to release a follicle, or sac, that contains an egg. The luteinizing hormone (LH) causes the ovaries to release a mature egg.

When the hormones are not strong enough to do their jobs, cysts can form, either inside your ovaries or outside of your ovaries. The eggs never "grow up" enough to be released from the nest, so to speak, and so there is no ovulation and no menstruation. These sacs are referred to as cysts. In turn, the ovaries produce lower levels of estrogen and progesterone and increased levels of androgens.

The increased levels of androgen cause fewer menstrual cycles, so a vicious circle is created.

There is nothing simple about this diagnosis. Even the name seems to cause confusion. First, PCOS is not a disorder that only affects your ovaries. It affects your entire endocrine system, especially your pancreas. Second, some women may be diagnosed with PCOS despite the absence of cysts on or in their ovaries. In light of this, The National Institutes of Health has recommended that the name of the syndrome be changed to one that reflects the metabolic, psychological, and reproductive problems that arise as a result of this syndrome.

There are other confusing issues regarding PCOS. Although PCOS is often associated with weight and the assumption that PCOS is caused by obesity or being overweight is a common one, women of all shapes and sizes are diagnosed with it. According to Natalia Lusinski, a reporter who has written about PCOS for *Bustle*, some women are told that if they lose weight, their infertility can be cured, but this is not necessarily true. Lusinski also says that some women are told that a hysterectomy will cure their PCOS. This is also a falsehood, since PCOS is an endocrine disorder.

Who Is Affected by PCOS?

Any woman who has started ovulating and menstruating, and has not yet reached menopause, is at risk for PCOS. However, the disorder typically affects women who are between the ages of fifteen and forty-four. It is estimated that between two and twenty-six percent of the female population is affected by PCOS.

Usually, the syndrome appears during puberty. Most women are diagnosed during their teens and early twenties. Although it is uncommon, some women receive their PCOS diagnosis in their thirties or forties.

Some women do not even realize they have PCOS, which is why there is such a huge gap in the percentages of those affected. According to one study, seventy percent of women who have PCOS are not aware of it. That is a significant number of the population who are unknowingly suffering from a treatable disorder.

There are a few reasons why women who suffer from PCOS have not received a proper diagnosis. One of the most frightening facts about PCOS is that some women have to wait two or more years for a diagnosis. Some women have to visit several doctors before a true diagnosis is found. There are several reasons for both of these problems.

The first reason is that women may seek treatment for the symptoms, unaware of the root cause of the problem. For example, a woman with excessive acne may visit a dermatologist to treat the skin condition, not knowing that the underlying cause is excessive amounts of androgens.

One woman stated that when her hair started thinning, she thought that since her mother and her aunts also had suffered through thinning hair, that it was just genetic. She was right about the fact that it was genetic. However, the cause of her thinning hair was PCOS. It was a very long time before all of her symptoms were added up together to come up with an accurate diagnosis.

Another reason why women are undiagnosed is that the process can take a very long time—even years. Because there is not one single test that can be done to determine whether you have PCOS, the doctors must conduct a battery of tests, analyze the results, and then rule out any other potential health issues that might be causing similar signs and symptoms.

Women may also be embarrassed to talk about their problems. It may be difficult for a woman to discuss the fact that she has irregular periods or extremely heavy periods.

Unfortunately, there is another reason why some women are not diagnosed with PCOS until later. The fact is, many doctors are simply not conscious of the disorder and tend to diagnose the symptoms, as opposed to the actual disorder. Some doctors may actually blame the woman for her symptoms. In Lusinski's article, where several women who suffer from PCOS were interviewed, Nikki stated that when she first went to the doctor to try to figure out what was wrong with her, he accused her of being a secret eater and gave her medication for diabetes. Every time Nikki went back, the doctor accused her of being a secret eater, even when she was not eating at all. Then, he simply increased her diabetes medication, which made her sick.

What Causes PCOS?

Doctors are not sure what causes PCOS. As reported by Lusinski, Kaitlin stated that she tried a lot of different treatments for her PCOS that didn't work. When she went back to her doctor seeking answers, Kaitlin was told they didn't know what caused her PCOS. Kaitlin said, "You can imagine how frustrating that can be when this syndrome affects you on so many levels."

Though we don't know the exact cause of PCOS right now, there is hope for the future. There are a lot of health experts in the field who are aware that more information is needed and are conducting studies to help determine causes and develop treatments.

One of the main indications of PCOS is increased levels of androgens or male hormones. The question is: What causes women to have higher than normal levels of testosterone?

One thing is for certain: Obesity does not cause PCOS. Obese, overweight, and lean women all suffer from PCOS. Take this experience shared by one woman named Holly. She was told that she could not have PCOS because she was not overweight. Skeptical of her doctor's assessment, Holly got a second opinion, which confirmed that her instincts were right. She was diagnosed with PCOS.

Lusinski also identified two other women who were told by their doctors they were eating too much and not exercising enough. They were told this was the reason for their irregular periods.

Higher Levels of Male Hormones

The high levels of the male hormone prevent ovulation, which causes the sacs, or cysts, to gather in the ovaries. Research indicates that the higher levels of testosterone interfere with the female hormones that develop and release the eggs. However, doctors are not sure why some women produce higher levels of androgens. One possible culprit is insulin resistance.

In addition to contributing to PCOS, higher levels of testosterone cause women to grow a lot of hair on their faces, chests, butts, necks, arms, legs, and bellies. It may also cause scalp hair to thin and even male pattern baldness.

Laura Starr, who was diagnosed with PCOS when she was sixteen, said that the additional facial hair made her feel very self-conscious. People would often tell her that she had something on her chin. That "something" was facial hair and this would cause her great embarrassment. Speaking with ABC News, she shared that now she feels comfortable enough to be around her family and friends with the excessive hair growth, but she feels as though she must shave or wax anytime she goes out in public.

Hormone Imbalance

The hormone imbalance causes two significant issues for women with PCOS. The first issue is irregular menstrual cycles. Women typically have between ten and seventeen periods each year. Women with PCOS have six to eight periods each year, or even fewer. If they do have a period, it may be extremely light because no ovulation has occurred. On the flip side, their periods may have an extremely heavy flow, because the uterine lining has been building up continuously. The cycles may also be longer. Instead of a twenty-eight-day cycle, women with PCOS may have cycles that last between thirty-two and thirty-six days.

Infertility is another issue that is caused by a hormonal imbalance. If an egg is not released from the ovaries, then a baby cannot be conceived. According to the American College of Obstetricians and Gynecologists, PCOS is the leading cause of infertility in women. Approximately eighty percent of women who suffer from PCOS are infertile. However, there are treatments that can be used to increase fertility.

Insulin Resistance

Insulin resistance is another possible cause of PCOS. Around seventy percent of women who suffer from PCOS are insulin resistant. This means that their bodies are unable to use insulin properly. The body is not able to send enough sugars to the cells that need glucose for energy.

To compensate, the body produces even more insulin. The extra insulin produces increased levels of male hormones. In addition, the extra insulin can shut down ovarian function.

While obesity is a significant contributor to insulin resistance, it is not the only cause. There are women with lean body type who are insulin resistance.

An additional effect of insulin resistance is skin changes, such as thickening and darkening of patches of skin.

Inflammation

A third potential cause of PCOS may be inflammation in the body. Obesity is a significant cause of inflammation.

Genetic Links

Doctors agree that PCOS seems to run in families. Researchers believe there are many genes involved, not just one.

A New Study Identifies One Potential Cause

French scientist Paolo Giacobini and his associates have discovered that PCOS may be caused before you are even born. The scientists discovered that thirty percent of women who have PCOS have higher levels of the anti-Mullerian hormone. These women would have been exposed to higher levels of this hormone while they were still in the womb.

Because PCOS tends to run in families, the scientists wanted to find out if the imbalance of this hormone would cause the daughters to be affected. After conducting several experiments with mice, they determined that the increased levels of the hormone had a direct effect on the daughters.

The study was important because, not only did it establish a potential cause for PCOS, but it also led to a potential treatment, and even a cure, for the syndrome. Scientists will begin studies of a drug called Cetrorelix on women who suffer from PCOS. Previous studies of the drug on mice indicate that it can effectively reverse the symptoms of PCOS.

This study may also explain why women who suffer from PCOS find it easier to get pregnant when they are older. Women tend to decrease hormone production as they age, particularly the anti-Mullerian hormone.

What Are the Symptoms of PCOS?

Do you have symptoms of PCOS but have not been diagnosed yet? You are not alone. More than seventy percent of women who suffer from PCOS do not realize it. They simply suffer in silence.

How do you know if you are a part of that seventy percent? There are early warning signs and symptoms of PCOS that you can be aware of. If you notice these signs, then there are several tests that your doctors can use to determine whether you may be affected by PCOS.

Just like with every other illness, syndrome, and disease, you may not have all of the symptoms. However, there are some early warning signs of PCOS, and even if you have just one of them, you should talk to your doctor. This is especially true if your menstrual cycles are irregular.

Early Warning Signs

There are several warning signs that can signal that you should check in with a doctor about a possible PCOS diagnosis.

1. Do you have extremely heavy periods, irregular periods, or no periods at all? The hormone imbalance caused by PCOS, especially the increased male hormones, can mess with your menstrual cycle.

    a. Heavy periods occur because there is an extra build-up of the uterine lining when it is not released regularly. It is extremely important to talk to a doctor about this, because the build-up of the uterine lining can lead to an increased risk of developing endometrial cancer.

    b. Irregular periods are caused when immature eggs are not released. Instead, they stay in their sacs within the ovaries. These sacs are the cysts that accumulate. Because mature eggs are not released, you may find it difficult to become pregnant.

    c. No periods are caused when there are no eggs that develop to maturity. This means the body does not release any eggs at all. Instead, they build up in your ovaries. Because the body releases no eggs, you become infertile.

2. Have you tried, and failed, to get pregnant? This could be an early warning sign of PCOS. It is very

difficult to become pregnant when mature eggs are not ovulated during regular cycles.

3. Repeated miscarriages may also signify PCOS. The extra hormones produced may make it difficult for a baby to survive.

4. Weight gain is another sign of PCOS, especially weight gain around the belly.

5. Difficulty losing weight could indicate PCOS.

Symptoms

In addition to the early warning signs of PCOS, there are many other symptoms that may be present.

1. Pelvic pain may result from the cysts that are accumulating in your ovaries. You may also have as many as twenty-five cysts that are attached to the outside of an ovary. Another cause of pelvic pain is the uterine lining growth, which is not shed due to a lack of menstruation. However, health care professionals state that many women do not feel any pelvic pain. They refer to ovarian cysts as the "silent symptom" because many women do not feel them.

2. Approximately seventy percent of the women who suffer from PCOS experience hirsutism, or extra hair growth on the face and other body parts, such as the chest, belly, back, and butt. This is another warning sign that you might be affected by the extra androgen produced by your ovaries. The testosterone stimulates the hair follicles in these areas.

3. Very oily skin and/or excessive acne on your face,

chest, and back may indicate PCOS. This is especially true if the acne is not cleared up by regular treatments.

4. Thinning hair or male pattern baldness may be caused by the excess production of androgen.

5. Patches of thick, dark skin around your neck, breast, and groin areas may be caused by the insulin resistance associated with PCOS. Skin tags, especially under your arms or on your neck, may be caused by insulin resistance.

Do Not Ignore Your Body's Warning

A lot of women may brush off the symptoms as being nothing. Others opt to "just deal with it."

You shouldn't have to "just deal" with the discomforts caused by PCOS. These discomforts and inconveniences can turn into something a lot more serious. There are long-term health complications that can be caused by PCOS.

Dr. Amy Schutt describes PCOS as "the canary in the coal mine" because it is often a warning for other, serious health conditions, such as prediabetes, insulin resistance, and uterine abnormalities. "Women with PCOS are at risk in the future of developing type 2 diabetes, metabolic syndrome, uterine cancer, and possible heart disease. So it is very important that we identify PCOS when women are young and when we can best intervene."

Approximately eighty percent of women who suffer from PCOS must also deal with weight gain. The additional weight is usually stored in the belly area and increases the risk for type 2 diabetes and metabolic syndrome. While weight gain does not cause PCOS, research indicates that women who lose be-tween two and ten percent of their weight can improve their symptoms.

Diabetes is one possible complication of PCOS. Women who suffer from PCOS have four times the risk of receiving a diagnosis of type 2 diabetes than women who do not. Approx-imately fifty percent of women with PCOS will develop type 2 diabetes before they are forty years old. Between five and fif-teen percent of women with PCOS will develop type 2 dia-betes within three years of their diagnosis.

Metabolic Syndrome is a combination of high blood pres-sure and high cholesterol, which increases the risk of heart disease. Women who suffer from PCOS have higher levels of bad cholesterol (LDL), and lower levels of good cholesterol (HDL). They also have a higher risk of developing high blood pressure and stiff or clogged arteries. This is especially true if type 2 diabetes is not well managed.

Endometrial cancer is another concern for women who suffer from PCOS. With normal menstruation, the uterine lin-ing is shed. However, when there is no menstruation, the lin-ing simply builds up. There is a constant estrogen stimulation to the lining, but there is no protection from progesterone. As the cells in the endometrium continue to bunch together, they begin to take abnormal forms, which leads to cancer. Studies indicate that women with PCOS are three times more likely to develop endometrial cancer than women who do not suffer from the syndrome.

Sleep apnea is yet another issue for women who suffer from PCOS. Sleep apnea occurs when there are pauses in the breath-ing process while sleeping. It is estimated that women with

PCOS are thirty times more likely than other women to have sleep apnea. Not only does sleep apnea increase fatigue, but it can also lead to an increased risk for type 2 diabetes and high blood pressure.

Depression and anxiety are also associated with PCOS. Studies indicate that women who suffer from PCOS are three times as likely to have depression, anxiety, or bipolar disorder. Although health experts do not know specifically why this is true, they speculate that it could be due, in part, to hormonal imbalances and higher amounts of androgens. These mental health issues may also form as a result of these women being forced to deal with things like infertility, baldness, and excessive hair. Fatigue, caused by sleep disorders that are associated with PCOS, may contribute to depression and anxiety.

Eating Disorders become an issue for women who are obsessed with their weight. Women who try any means to lose weight may develop anorexia nervosa or bulimia. Unfortunately, eating disorders only create additional health problems and, in some cases, can lead to death.

Nonalcoholic Steatohepatitis is an inflammation in the liver that is not caused by alcohol consumption. Two of the causes of this disease are obesity and insulin resistance which are common factors with women who suffer from PCOS.

Miscarriages and premature births are among other common issues that women who suffer from PCOS face. There are several potential reasons for this, including excessive androgens and excessive insulin.

Doctor's Examination

Unfortunately, there is no such thing as a "PCOS test." Different major health organizations have different criteria that is used to determine whether a person has PCOS. Some groups say that a diagnosis can be made if it is determined that the woman has higher than normal levels of the male hormones. Other health organizations state that the high levels of the male hormones must be present but must be accompanied by irregular ovulation. Others still suggest that a diagnosis can be made if the woman has two out of three significant symptoms: high male hormone levels, cysts on the ovaries, and irregular menstruation.

This means that actually receiving a diagnosis can be time-consuming and frustrating because the doctor has to analyze a bunch of different health issues.

The doctor analyzes different aspects of your health to determine whether you are suffering from PCOS, or if you are affected by a different health issue that has similar symptoms. A diagnosis of PCOS is made after all other possible issues have been eliminated.

Once you arrive at your doctor's office with a list of your symptoms, there are several ways to determine whether you suffer from PCOS.

When you first visit with the doctor, he or she will have questions for you about your menstrual cycle. The doctor will want to know about regularity and also about your flow, as a significantly heavy flow can indicate problems for you. In addition, the doctor will have other questions about your health, such as whether you suffer from headaches and whether you are struggling with weight management.

The doctor will also want to know whether other people in your family have similar problems, especially any sisters, aunts, your mother, or grandmother.

You will also have a physical. The doctor will check your skin to determine whether you have any of the tell-tale thick, dark skin marks that indicate higher levels of the male hormone. Your body mass index (BMI) will also be measured, as well as your waist size. The doctor will also check to determine whether you have excessive hair on your face, chest, belly, or butt. In addition, you will be examined for excessive acne.

The doctor may do a pelvic exam to check your ovaries and order an ultrasound to get a closer look at your ovaries. It is important to note that even if you have cysts in or on your ovaries, you may not receive a diagnosis of PCOS. By the same token, you may have PCOS even if there are no cysts.

A blood test may be conducted to determine blood sugar levels and hormone levels.

Going back to Lusinski's article, another woman featured was Regina who said that she was frustrated because when she went to the doctor about her symptoms, she was told by the doctor that she did not have PCOS because there were no cysts on her ovaries. Regina was forgiving of the doctor but said it taught her a valuable lesson that she had to be aware and informed, and that she had to take charge of her own condition. She did this by finding a different doctor.

Making a diagnosis of PCOS can be difficult and time-consuming. Professor Helena Teede, from Monash University in Australia, is a leading expert on PCOS. According to her, part of the problem is that PCOS is so complex, and doctors have a hard time wrapping their heads around how to find a diagnosis. The Polycystic Ovary Syndrome Association of Australia is working with Monash University to find a way to make a diagnosis "clearer and simpler."

Do Not Give Up

Amy Medling, the founder of PCOSdiva.com, encourages women to channel their inner "diva" when seeking treatment. This requires being insistent that the doctor takes a look at all of your symptoms. If your doctor doesn't come up with a satisfactory answer, then get a second opinion or third opinion. Don't stop until you feel heard. With PCOS, you may have to become your own health advocate until you can find the right doctor who will work for you. Medling says that when you see the doctor, you must be honest and tell them all of your symptoms. She also stresses that you need to be assertive when getting lab tests, because the more information you have, the quicker you will be able to diagnose your condition and get a treatment plan started.

Discussions Surrounding the Diagnosis of PCOS

An international consortium led by the Centre for Research Excellence in PCOS, including thirty-seven PCOS professional societies and organizations from seventy-one countries, recently met to discuss issues surrounding PCOS, including the diagnosis of the syndrome. One of the recommendations from the consortium was that a diagnosis of PCOS should be made if a woman's menstrual cycle is not regular and if blood tests reveal that the woman has large amounts of male hormones. The consortium concluded an ultrasound of the ovaries is not needed to diagnose the syndrome since ultrasounds that pick up ovarian cysts may lead to a misdiagnosis. For instance, a woman might be diagnosed with PCOS while the true culprit is another issue, such as polycystic ovarian morphology (PCOM).

The consortium also stated that although Anti Mullerian hormones are connected to PCOS, the hormone levels cannot be used for diagnosis. They did not provide a reason for this.

While insulin resistance is considered to be a key feature of PCOS, the consortium determined that the measurement of insulin or blood sugar levels should not be used for diagnosis. High insulin levels can be a sign of many different health issues, like diabetes, so it cannot be reliably used for diagnostic purposes for PCOS.

More Research Is Needed

Although the medical community has known about PCOS for centuries, there is still a tremendous lack of information about the syndrome, the causes, effects, treatments, and perhaps a cure.

Professor Teede says it best: "What has been a really clear message from women is they are getting inadequate care, and then from health professionals that they're finding diagnosis difficult. One of the reasons is because we still don't fully understand the condition."

Since the international health community and PCOS experts are noticing that more and more women are being diagnosed with PCOS, we can only hope that a lot more research will be conducted. We can hope that soon doctors, scientists, and health advocates will a cure so women no longer have to deal with the symptoms, and have a less stressful, healthier life.

Chapter Summary

- PCOS affects approximately one-fourth of women in the United States.

- Many of the women who suffer from PCOS have not been diagnosed.

- There are many early warning signs and symptoms that should not be ignored.

- It is important that women who suffer from PCOS get treatment because the syndrome can develop into potentially life-threatening ailments.

In the next chapter, you will learn about the mental and emotional health associated with PCOS.

Chapter Two: The Hidden Symptom, Mental and Emotional Health With PCOS

With all of the symptoms, pain, worry, and stress women with PCOS face, it is not surprising that depression and anxiety accompany PCOS.

Women who were interviewed by ABC News said that their doctors simply did not believe there was anything wrong. Two women had to prove their cases to their doctors before they were taken seriously. Peggy, a woman who experienced this kind of frustrating push back from doctors, told ABC News, "People don't understand what I am feeling and medical professionals are unable or unwilling to offer help."

In addition to feeling unheard by medical professionals, another important contributor to the mental and emotional struggle is having to deal with the possibility of not being able to have children. Many women feel devastated when they learn having a baby may be difficult or impossible because of their PCOS. As you will learn in chapter seven, this is not the case for most women.

Because there are few guidelines regarding the diagnosis of PCOS, mental and emotional health are often overlooked. However, this is starting to change. At the consortium mentioned in chapter one, the members recommended that those diagnosed with PCOS should also be screened for mental and emotional health issues.

Several studies indicate that women with PCOS are three times more likely to be diagnosed with mental health disorders such as bipolar, obsessive-compulsive disorder, depression, and anxiety, as well as eating disorders. The symptoms are more likely to be severe. It was found that the children of mothers with PCOS were more likely to be diagnosed with ADHD or were more likely to be on the autism spectrum.

A study conducted by Cardiff University on seventeen hundred women diagnosed with PCOS found that more than twenty-three percent suffered from depression, more than eleven percent suffered from anxiety, and more than three percent suffered from bipolar disorder.

With all of that said, if you are diagnosed with PCOS, getting screened for mental health issues is a good idea.

Causes and Possible Solutions

There are several possible causes for the mental and emotional health issues that are associated with PCOS. Experts have not yet reached a mutual agreement on why women may suffer from these disorders, although they have named several potential contributors.

This begs the question: "If medical experts do not know why I am depressed, feeling anxious, or have mood swings, how are they going to help me overcome them?"

Obesity and Poor Body Image

ABC surveyed two hundred fifty women with PCOS. Approximately seventy percent of the women said they suffered from depression. More than twenty-five percent of the women attributed the cause of their depression to their weight or self-esteem issues.

For example, one woman who was diagnosed with PCOS said, "I feel like a big fat stack of shit." Another woman said, "I feel like a hairy, ugly, moody defect. I don't feel sexy or beautiful—I just want to be like other girls." Other women report that they suffer from self-hatred.

Studies have shown that people who are obese and have an increased risk of suffering from mental and emotional health issues. Although not every woman who suffers from PCOS is obese, there is an increased risk of obesity to be wary of.

Women who suffer from PCOS are eighty percent more likely to gain weight and have difficulty shedding the weight. This can lead to developing a poor body image. Pop culture can make this even worse because of the way they portray beautiful women. Having a negative body image can cause depression and anxiety and may even lead to the development of eating disorders like anorexia or bulimia.

For women with PCOS, it is important to work toward having a more positive body image. This does not mean that you have to be completely happy with your body at all times. It means that you do not have to allow your body image to keep you from having a happy life.

One way to develop a better body image is to understand that the images of women portrayed in media are not always realistic. It has even been said that after publishers, advertisers, and photographers are done manipulating the images, some models do not even recognize themselves. For example, any type of blemish is often photoshopped out. Some editors make the models' waists smaller and their chests bigger.

Understand that you are beautiful as you are. No two women are built the same. It is also important to understand that Barbie does not exist, and it is not possible to have a Barbie body. This means that you have to be realistic about your body type. Some women naturally are thin. Other women are not, and it is not possible for them to achieve a very lean look. And that is okay. Some of the most beautiful women in Hollywood have larger frames, such as Camryn Meinham (*Ghost Whisperer, The Practice*), Kirsten Vangsness (*Criminal Minds),* and Melissa McCarthy (*Ghostbusters, Spy, Gilmore Girls).*

Eliminate negative self-talk. Do not allow yourself to be rude and disrespectful to yourself. When you begin saying or thinking those negative comments, recognize that you are, and then force yourself to stop them. It will take some practice, but you can change your negative self talk to positive self-talk.

Focus on your positive attributes. Unless you are the Wicked Witch of the West and are the meanest, most hardhearted person in the world, you have some wonderful attributes. Focus on them. Focus on your kindness, your intelligence, and your determination. Focus on your beautiful eyes and appreciate that you have curves. Understand that you are beautiful.

Know When to Get Help

There comes a point when it's time to seek professional help, when the stress and the struggle are too difficult to manage on your own. But how do you know when it's time to seek help? Here are a few signs to look out for:

- When your negative self-talk becomes extreme. You have convinced yourself that you are hideous. That your image is awful.

- When your negative body image prevents you from engaging in the activities you used to love, including hanging out with friends and family.

- When you go on extreme diets to try to lose weight.

- When you begin an extreme exercise regime to try and lose weight.

- When you have unrealistic expectations for yourself. Even if you are able to lose forty pounds, you are not going to be able to do so overnight.

Body Issues Besides Weight Gain

Some of the physical symptoms, in addition to weight gain, that result from PCOS may also cause a negative body image. According to the media and many cultural expectations, women are supposed to have lustrous head hair and have no body hair. Yet the higher levels of male hormones can cause hair to thin or even male pattern baldness. In addition, the hormones may cause excessive body hair, including facial hair, which can be very embarrassing.

Acne can also become a problem. Patches of thick, dark skin may appear inconspicuous places. Skin tags, while not as noticeable, may also appear. These physical symptoms can make a woman feel very self-conscious about her appearance, which can create a negative body image.

There are some ways that these issues can be addressed. Hats, scarves, or wigs can help cover up thinning hair or baldness. Plucking and waxing hair can eliminate some of the excessive body hair. However, it might prove to be very difficult to eliminate all of the physical manifestations of the PCOS.

Excessive facial hair may be a huge contributor to a negative body image. If you are tired of plucking and waxing, laser hair removal might be a solution.

Seek Help When Needed

Just like with weight issues, you must recognize when you need to seek help with negative body issues related to the physical manifestations of your PCOS. Here are some warning signs that you may be struggling and in need of professional help:

1. When your negative self-talk is extreme and sincere.
2. When your negative body image prevents you from taking part in the activities you love, or when it interferes with your relationships with family and friends.
3. When you have unrealistic expectations for yourself.

Increased Insulin Resistance

Studies regarding whether increased insulin resistance causes mental and emotional health issues are inconclusive. Some studies indicate that there is a link between the two, while other studies indicate that there is no link. One study showed that there is a possible link between insulin resistance and higher anxiety levels. However, more research is needed to conclusively determine whether there is a link between the two.

If insulin resistance does contribute to mental and emotional issues, then there are medications that can help ease the symptoms, such as Metformin.

Hormone Imbalance

There is a known connection to hormones and mental and emotional health. However, there have not been enough studies conducted to determine whether higher levels of androgens in women can cause depression and anxiety. One study determined that there was no correlation between higher levels of testosterone and depression and anxiety. Another study indicated that there is a link between DHEAS, a type of androgen hormone, and an increased risk of depression and anxiety. Like many other issues associated with PCOS, more research is needed.

Chemicals in the Brain

There has been a long-time connection between chemicals in the brain and mental and emotional disorders. Neurotransmitters are chemicals that send messages in the brain and nervous system. Women who suffer from PCOS may have lower levels of neurotransmitters, such as serotonin (a neurotransmitter associated with positive feelings).

Infertility

Infertility is a common problem with women suffering from PCOS. When a woman is trying to get pregnant but is unable to, she can become discouraged, depressed, and feel anxious about whether she will be able to have children.

A Combination of Issues

Just as PCOS is a complicated syndrome, with a combination of symptoms and health effects, it is very likely that the increased depression seen in women who suffer from the syndrome is also caused by a combination of issues.

Treatment

Dealing with the symptoms of PCOS is hard enough. And there is no shame in experiencing depression, anxiety, and other mental and emotional health disorders. It is extremely important that you seek treatment for them. There are many different ways that a therapist, psychologist, or psychiatrist might treat your illnesses.

Cognitive Behavioral Therapy

Cognitive behavior therapy (CBT) is a talk therapy that may be used alone or used in combination with medications. Research has shown that CBT can help with depression, anxiety, sleep disorders, eating disorders, obsessive-compulsive disorder, and bipolar disorder, among others.

Cognitive behavior therapy is a goal-oriented approach to helping you with your mental and emotional health issues. The therapy asks you to focus on the specific issues you are facing. The therapist may ask you to do homework. You might be asked to read certain articles or practice what you have learned during sessions while you go about your daily life.

There are four steps in CBT. The first step is to identify what situations are presenting challenges to you. In your case, it could be dealing with the PCOS and the symptoms that accompany it such as weight gain, excessive hair, and infertility and even how it affects your relationships with other people. Then, you will work with your therapist to decide what specific goals you want to work on.

The second step is for you to become aware of your emotions, thoughts, and beliefs about the issues you are facing. For example, if you have a negative body image because of the physical symptoms of PCOS, then you will talk about your thoughts. This may include what you tell yourself about your problem (self-talk), your beliefs about yourself, other people, and situations. You may be encouraged to keep a journal and write down your thoughts and feelings as you go through your day.

Third, you will be asked to identify inaccurate or negative feelings about the situation. Your therapist will ask you to pay attention to your reactions around how you respond to different situations. For example, if you look in the mirror and see the facial hair, what does your body do? What thoughts about yourself go through your mind? How do you feel?

The fourth step in CBT is to determine whether your self-talk and the perceptions you have of yourself and your situation are based on fact or inaccurate perceptions. For example, if you are facing infertility, the therapist might ask you to determine whether your condition is your fault or if it is due to circumstances beyond your control. Did you truly purposefully give yourself the hormone condition that made ovulation difficult? Of course you did not. Does your infertility make you less of a woman? Of course not. At this point, you learn to replace the negative and inaccurate self-talk with the more accurate positive talk. You are as much a woman as every other female in this world. With treatment, it is possible that you can successfully conceive and give birth. When you practice positive self-talk and accurate thinking, it will become easier.

Many therapists prefer to use CBT because it will help you identify your challenges, such as depression, anxiety, and even the reasons why you might suffer from an eating disorder. Once you have identified your mental and emotional disorders and the reasons behind them, the therapist can help you discover ways to overcome them.

Another reason why CBT is preferred is because it is a very structured therapy session, and many people are able to combat their challenges with fewer sessions.

Cognitive-behavioral therapy has proven to help people with many aspects of mental and emotional issues, including:

1. Learning how to cope with chronic health problems (such as PCOS), including the symptoms associated with the syndrome.
2. Preventing a relapse of mental health symptoms. Because CBT helps you recognize the mental and emotional health issues that you are facing and what the symptoms are, you will be able to recognize the signs that might indicate you are heading down a negative path. For example, if you begin with the negative self-talk, you can recognize it, challenge the talk, and use positive self-talk to combat it.
3. Treat mental health issues when medications are not a good option. This can be especially important if you are trying to get pregnant, are pregnant, or are breastfeeding.
4. Learn how to manage your emotions. You know you are sad, depressed, or have low self-esteem. Cognitive behavior therapy can help you recognize the

emotions, the signs, and help you learn tools to overcome them.

It is important to understand that once you begin CBT, you will not have instant results. Like all things in life, you have to work on it. You have to practice the techniques. It may not cure your anxiety or depression. However, it will give you tools that you can use to work through negative situations and feelings.

Lifestyle Changes

Lifestyle changes are recommended for many issues surrounding PCOS. This includes including healthy levels of exercise and a healthy diet.

Exercise

Research has shown that people who suffer from anxiety and depression have fewer symptoms if they exercise at least a hundred and fifty minutes per week. Harvard Health suggests that exercise can alleviate symptoms related to depression and anxiety unless those disorders are particularly severe.

When you exercise, your body releases the positive or "feel good" endorphins, which are hormones that improve your mood and sense of well-being. Brain scans show that the hippocampus part of the brain, which regulates mood, is smaller in people who are depressed. However, exercise stimulates the cell growth in that part of the brain so that it can help stabilize your moods, and decrease your depression.

Exercising can also help take your mind off the issues that are causing you stress or anxiety. It allows you the opportunity to escape from the negative and inaccurate thoughts that feed your anxiety and depression.

The Mayo Clinic lists several other benefits of exercise that can help improve your mental and emotional symptoms. Here are a few big ones:

1. Exercising can help you gain confidence. When you make a goal to get into an exercise regime, and then you keep your goal, you'll feel a sense of accomplishment that can boost your self-image. Getting into shape can make you feel better about your appearance as well. The added benefit is that it can help you lose a bit of weight, which can result in reduced insulin resistance and reduced risk for developing metabolic syndrome.

2. Exercise can help improve social interactions. Join a gym, fitness class, or recreational sports team. These group-based activities give you the opportunity to interact with people who have similar goals to yours. If group activities seem intimidating at first, start small and work your way up. Even something as simple as taking a walk around the block may give you the chance to interact with others by exchanging waves or smiles.

3. Exercise is a healthy coping mechanism. Exercise gives you the opportunity to release your fears, frustrations, anger, and other negative feelings in a healthy way. It also gives you an opportunity to walk away from a problem and see it from a different perspective. Many times when you focus on a problem for too long, you get stuck in a rut. When you walk away from the problem, you give yourself

the opportunity to think about something else, and then you can approach the problem from another angle. Exercising gives you the opportunity to come up with possible solutions.

Depression can make it hard to feel motivated. Even tackling simple chores can be a challenge. You may also lose interest in activities that you enjoy. So, something like starting a new exercise regime can feel like an impossible task. Be kind and patient with yourself. Start small and build from there. Here are a few strategies that can help:

1. Take a five-minute walk. If you feel comfortable, add on more time. Challenge yourself to walk at least five minutes per day.
2. You do not have to jog, go to the gym every day, or take part in rigorous activities. Choose an activity you enjoy. It can be walking around the block, a swim in the pool, yoga, or any other activity that gets your body moving.
3. Make sure you set reasonable goals. For example, while a goal of losing ten pounds a week is totally unrealistic, a goal of losing one pound per week is achievable and safe. Your goals can be challenging, but they must be attainable.
4. Approach exercising as something you enjoy doing, not something that must be done. If you view exercise as a chore, then you are less likely to continue engaging in that activity. However, if you consider it to be an activity that you enjoy doing, then you are

more likely to follow through with them.

5. Analyze any barriers that would prevent you from creating a successful exercise routine. If you do not feel comfortable exercising in public spaces, then create a routine at home. If high-intensity workouts are too challenging for your skill level, do low impact aerobics. Use what you have available like stairs or soup cans to substitute for hand weights. Think outside the box.

6. Understand that you will face setbacks and obstacles in your plans. You might skip a day. That does not mean you are lazy or that you cannot get back on track. It means that you skipped a day, and you will pick up where you left off.

7. Make sure that you give yourself credit for every accomplishment, regardless of how small you think it is.

Like all other treatments, you might not notice an immediate change. Over time, the positive effects will accumulate, and you will notice a decrease in your depression and anxiety symptoms. It is important to remember that you must continue exercising even after you start to feel better in order to sustain the positive effects.

Diet

Although there are many foods that can help with depression, anxiety, and other mental and emotional health issues, studies have found that there is no correlation between low-calorie diets and long-term relief of symptoms. One study indicated that low-calorie diets did not improve symptoms of anxiety and only improved symptoms from depression for a short time.

Eating foods that are high in omega-3 fatty acids may also relieve symptoms of depression and anxiety. Sardines, herring, wild salmon, and farmed oysters are a good source of omega-3 fatty acids. Canola oil and soybean oil also have fatty acids in them. Walnuts, tofu, and leafy green vegetables are also a good source of omega-3 fatty acids. You can also take fish oil supplements, either by themselves or with vitamin D, which can increase your levels of fatty acids.

Smart carbs are another food group that may help increase serotonin levels. Research has indicated that there is a link between a craving for carbohydrates and depression. You can still have carbs and eat a healthy diet. The key is to avoid processed carbs, like cakes and cookies. Fruits, vegetables, and nuts have carbohydrates that will satisfy your cravings. The bonus with these foods is that they are also high in fiber.

High protein foods have also shown to increase serotonin. Foods such as tuna, chicken, and turkey can help ease the symptoms of depression and anxiety. Beans, low-fat cheese, yogurt, lean beef, poultry, fish, peas, and soy foods have proteins that can help with depression.

Consuming foods that have high vitamin B content can also help with depression. Vitamin B12 has been shown to increase energy levels. Beans, nuts, most fruits, and dark green vegetables, as well as low-fat animal products and low-fat dairy products, have high amounts of these vitamins that can help you combat the symptoms of depression and anxiety.

Likewise, it is important to make sure that you get enough vitamin D. Foods that are high in vitamin D include salmon, sardines, herring, cod liver oil, tuna, oysters, shrimp, egg yolks, mushrooms, and fortified foods (such as vitamin D cow milk, soy milk, orange juice, cereal, and oatmeal).

Research has also found a link between depression and low selenium. Therefore, eating foods that have high selenium levels can help you overcome your depression and anxiety symptoms. Foods that include selenium include beans, nuts, lean meat, low-fat dairy products, seeds, seafood, and whole grains.

It is important to watch your caffeine intake as too much caffeine can cause anxiety. To make sure that you reduce sleeping issues, you should stop drinking caffeine around noon. It is also extremely important to avoid alcohol and drugs.

Like with obesity, there is a cycle between poor nutrition and depression. Poor nutrition can affect your body and brain chemistry, causing depression. However, people tend to engage in unhealthy eating habits when they are depressed. Therefore, to break the cycle it is exceedingly important that you eat healthily.

Sleep

Like with obesity and nutrition, there is a cycle with a lack of sleep and depression. Not getting enough sleep can't cause depression. However, many people who struggle with sleep issues tend to suffer from depression. Most health experts agree that adults need seven to nine hours of sleep each night. However, surveys indicate that most people get less than seven hours. Oversleeping is another indication of depression.

Sleep is when the body restores itself. A lack of restful sleep can cause you to be tense, irritable, and hyper-vigilant. A lack of sleep will eventually lead to fatigue, making it harder to keep up with regular physical activities, like working out. If you're exercising less frequently or not at all, you will likely experience an increase in symptoms of depression and anxiety.

If you struggle with insomnia, your doctor may recommend over the counter medications that can help you fall asleep, such as Unisom or Zzzquill. There are also prescription medications that can help you sleep.

Here are a few simple ways to treat your insomnia at home:

1. Meditation right before bed can help clear your mind of your negative thoughts. There are a lot of meditative techniques you can use to calm your mind.
2. Read a book before bed.
3. Listen to soft music with a slow tempo. Classical music is a popular choice.
4. Write a list of things you need to accomplish the next day so you're not thinking about them while you are trying to sleep.
5. Likewise, write a list of your worries right before you go to bed.
6. Avoid looking at computer screens, television screens, or phone screens right before bed. The bright light emitted from these technologies can prevent the release of melatonin, a hormone that tells your brain that it is time to sleep.
7. Practice yoga.
8. Practice breathing exercises to calm your body.
9. Avoid taking medications, eating food, or drinking liquids that contain caffeine for several hours before you try to sleep.

10. Do not simply lie in bed tossing and turning when you are unable to sleep. Get out of bed, go to another room. Read, or do some other light activity until you are drowsy, then go back to bed.

11. The bed should only be used for sleeping and sex. That way, when you go to bed, it is a signal to your body that it is time to sleep.

12. A warm shower before you go to bed will help you fall into a deep sleep as your body cools.

13. Keep your room temperature cool.

14. A white noise machine, or a machine that produces nature sounds, may help you block out other sounds that would keep you awake.

15. Blackout shades can help prevent outside lights from keeping you awake, as can a sleeping mask.

Medications

Many doctors will prescribe medications to help treat depression, anxiety, bipolar disorder, and many other mental and emotional illnesses. The medications work by balancing out the neurotransmitters in your brain that affect your moods and emotions, such as serotonin. The medications can help you sleep better, eat better, and make you more motivated to exercise and do the activities that you enjoy. This, in turn, helps combat the symptoms you are struggling with.

It is important to note, just like with all treatments, you will not notice an immediate effect. In fact, a lot of the medications do not take effect until four or five weeks after you take them. For the medications to work quicker, you have to take them as they are prescribed.

Another important aspect to note is that while approximately sixty percent of people will feel better with the first type of medication they take, others will need to try a different type of medication until they see results. Unfortunately, there is not a one size fits all approach to the type and dosage of medication needed to treat your symptoms.

Doctors may also prescribe multiple medications to treat different symptoms. For example, let's say the first medication you take is a mood stabilizer, and you feel a partial change, but your anxiety is still affecting you, then the doctor may add a medication that will help decrease your anxiety symptoms.

The most important thing to note when you are taking medications is that you must communicate with your doctor. Be completely honest about how you are feeling and how the medications are affecting you. After all, the ultimate goal for the medications is to alleviate your symptoms. When you talk to your mental health care professional, make sure that the person understands everything that you are feeling. There is nothing to be ashamed of, and the more information they have, the more likely an effective treatment can be recommended.

Yoga

There are many research studies that indicate that yoga can be a significant help in reducing depression, bipolar disorder, and anxiety. It improves energy levels and decreases stress levels. Yoga can be used to help reduce chronic pain, chronic illnesses and improve overall physical health.

Yoga helps you deal with their depression in two ways. First, it allows you to focus your mind on the present moment and to clear your mind of any negative thoughts. Movements that are controlled and focused can help create a connection between your body and your mind.

Yoga focuses on gentle and calming motions. The poses are flexible, so everyone can participate in each pose. Yoga focuses on smooth movements, breathing exercises, and concentration. In addition, yoga requires you to focus on positive images designed to calm your body and your mind.

Practicing yoga can help reduce your resting heart rate, lower your blood pressure, help ease your breathing, increase pain tolerance, and decrease stress.

The other great thing about practicing yoga is that you can join a studio, practice one on one with an instructor, or practice at home, alone, with instructional videos. There are many different poses that target specific issues such as relaxation, increasing blood flow throughout the body, and finding proper body alignment.

Breathing Exercises

Breathing exercises are a great way to help alleviate symptoms of depression, anxiety, and bipolar disorder. When you are focused on your breathing, you are not focused as much on anything else, including stressful situations you are facing. You are simply focused on your breathing.

Many people tend to engage in shallow breathing, which can increase symptoms of depression and anxiety. Shallow breathing can cause your fight or flight instincts to kick in, which contributes to anxiety. On the other hand, breathing exercises, which includes deep breathing, stimulate your parasympathetic system and have the opposite effect. Deep breathing takes your body out of the fight or flight stage and into a calmer state.

Breathing exercises can lower blood pressure and regulate your heartbeat. This is especially useful if you are prone to anxiety attacks.

There are many breathing exercises that you can find online that can help reduce symptoms of depression and anxiety. Like many other "exercises" you may have to practice to get the hang of some of them.

Progressive Relaxation

Sit or lie down in a comfortable spot. While you are focused on breathing in and out with slow deep breaths, you will relax each one of your muscle groups. Start with your feet. Tense your muscles in your feet, and then completely relax them. Then, tense your calves, and completely relax them. Concentrating on your breathing, slowly move up your body until you have released the tension in all of your muscles.

Count of Four

This breathing technique requires you to focus on your breath, which dispels negative and stressful thoughts. Sit or lie down in a comfortable spot. Breathe out completely. Then breathe in through your nose to the count of four. Hold the breath for a count of four. Then exhale through your mouth to a count of four. Repeat until you feel a calmness settle in.

4-7-8 Technique

This technique requires you to lie down comfortably. Exhale completely through your mouth around your tongue, making a whooshing sound. Pursing your lips can help with this. Then close your mouth and inhale through your nose to a count of four. Hold your breath for a count to seven. Then exhale through your mouth, making the whooshing sound while counting to eight.

Experts recommend that you do not do this more than four times in one sitting.

Deep Breathing

Sit in a place where your entire body is completely supported. Breathe in deeply through your nose until you feel as though your belly is full of air. You should be able to see your belly rise as you breathe in. Then breathe out through your nose, watching your belly deflate.

Meditation

Research has indicated that mediation is a great way to handle stress, depression, and anxiety because meditation changes your reaction to those feelings. "Meditation trains the brain to achieve sustained focus, and to return to that focus when negative thinking, emotions, and physical sensations intrude—which happens a lot when you feel stressed and anxious," says Dr. John W. Denninger, director of research at the Benson-Henry Institute for Mind-Body Medicine at Harvard-affiliated Massachusetts General Hospital.

Studies have shown that meditation can actually change the specific areas of the brain that are specifically associated with depression. There are two brain regions that are associated with depression and anxiety. The medial prefrontal cortex becomes hyperactive in people who suffer from depression. This is the part of the brain that processes information about yourself, including worrying about yourself and thinking about the past. The amygdala is the "fear center" of your brain, which triggers the fight or flight response. These two brain regions feed off of each other to create depression and anxiety. Meditation helps to break the connection between these two brain sections.

Meditation helps you to ignore the feelings of stress and anxiety. In addition, meditation has been shown to increase the gray matter in the hippocampus, which then helps the hippocampus grow. As mentioned before, the hippocampus tends to shrink in depressed people.

The goal of meditation is not to eliminate negative thoughts and feelings. Instead, meditation helps you to learn that you do not have to act on these thoughts and feelings. You will learn to recognize that while you may have them, the thoughts and feelings are not who you are.

Meditation can also help you deal with stressful situations. For example, if you have a dentist's appointment, meditating before you go can help you achieve a state of calm.

The great thing about meditation is that there are several different techniques you can use. You can meditate anywhere. There is no specific amount of time you must spend meditating at one time, and there is no specific amount of time you must meditate per day or week. It is a very flexible technique that can be molded to fit into your life.

Get Started

1. Find a comfortable place to sit.
2. Set a time limit. Mindful.Com recommends that you should limit your first sessions to five or ten minutes until you get into the habit of meditating.
3. Notice your body and how it is positioned—whether you are sitting on your knees, cross-legged, or what have you.
4. Pay attention to your breathing. Focus on how you breathe in and breathe out.

5. Notice when your thoughts wander away from your breathing. Return your thoughts to your breathing.
6. Do not judge your mind or your thoughts. Simply notice that your thoughts have wandered.
7. When you are done meditating, notice your environment and any sights and sounds around you. Notice how you feel, and your thoughts and emotions.

There are many meditation techniques you can use, from body scanning to meditating while you walk. Meditation can help you control your stress and anxiety, regardless of where you are or what is going on around you.

Hobbies

Hobbies are a great way to help you deal with your stress, anxiety, and depression. When you are focused on activities that you enjoy, it helps take your mind off of the negative situations in your life.

Many hobbies are creative in one way or another. When you accomplish something, you feel successful. It can be anything from planting flowers, crocheting a blanket, or making a beautiful cake.

Many hobbies provide a positive outlet for stress. Someone who paints can unleash their negative emotions on the canvas. A person who makes cakes can turn their negative feelings into something beautiful and yummy.

Although many people find it hard to get started with any activity when they are depressed, including those they love, it is important that you take that first step. Just as with exercising, start small. Look at a recipe you want to try or a model airplane you want to build. The next step is to buy the ingredients or parts you need. Before you know it, your mind will be focused on enjoying the activity instead of cycling through negative thoughts.

Social Interactions

Depression and anxiety often cause isolation. However, it is very important to avoid cutting friends and family out of your life. Loved ones can provide a great support system.

Friends and family can even provide a welcome distraction to keep your mind off of negative and stressful situations. It is easier to go bowling, out to eat, or engage in other fun activities when you are around other people.

Know That You Are Not Alone

Although you may feel as though you are a tiny island, alone in a sea of women who do not have to deal with the painful, inconvenient, and difficult symptoms that you do, you are not alone.

Sharing your experience with others who understand your struggles can foster a sense of community and reducing feelings of loneliness and isolation. Rest assured, there are women out there who know firsthand what you're going through.

Support groups exist for exactly this reason. You can join support groups that are in your area and attend in person, or you can join online support groups. Not only do they give you the opportunity to talk about your illness, but they also provide a forum where you can trade tips on treatments that others have tried.

1. Women's Hair Loss Project - https://www.womenshairlossproject.com - A forum

where women share their stories and resources regarding the hair loss associated with PCOS.

2. Soul Cysters - http://www.soulcysters.net - is a forum where women can share their stories and talk to other people who suffer from PCOS.

3. My PCOS Team - https://www.mypcosteam.com - is an online social network that helps women provide emotional support to each other. It is also a place where women provide practical tips for how to deal with PCOS.

4. PCOS Diva - https://pcosdiva.com - A forum run by a woman who took control of her disease and her symptoms. She provides a lot of information on different ways you can do the same.

Chapter Summary

● Many women who suffer from PCOS also often suffer from mental and emotional disorders.

● The links between mental and emotional disorders are not known.

● There are a variety of ways you can work through mental and emotional disorders and get back to living.

In the next chapter, you will learn about what you need to know about reversing PCOS.

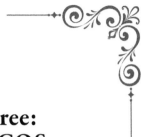

Chapter Three:
Reversing PCOS
and What You Need
to Know

F inding a treatment for PCOS can be just as frustrating as getting the initial diagnosis. Andrea, in Lusinksi's article, said it best: "The fact is that doctors have not really discovered exactly how to fix PCOS, and they insist on treating it solely as a reproductive issue, ignoring all of the endocrine/neurology aspects of this illness."

Although there is no known cure for PCOS at this time, ongoing research shows promising treatments that can control the causes and alleviate the symptoms. You do not have to simply bear the effects of PCOS. There is help for you.

First, it is important to note is that not all treatments and options will work the same for every woman. Just as the disorder affects women differently, the treatments will as well. It is very important that you talk to your doctor about any treatments, exercise programs, diets, or other options before you get started.

Quit Smoking

Are you a smoker? If you are, you should know that this habit is probably impacting your hormones. Studies indicate that there may be a link between nicotine and increased testosterone levels in women. There is also a correlation between smoking and increased insulin resistance.

There is a plethora of information and resources available for those who wish to quit smoking. Your doctor and the internet can be excellent starting points on your journey to quitting. While some people are able to quit cold turkey, most need a little extra help. Here are a few quitting strategies to explore:

1. Cigarette replacements, such as nicotine patches or gum.
2. E-cigarettes, which allow you to control the amount of nicotine you use. You can gradually decrease the amount of nicotine until you are weaned off.
3. Champix can be prescribed, which helps increase dopamine levels. Dopamine levels are often increased by smoking, so when people try to stop, they often feel depressed or anxious.
4. Bupropion is an antidepressant that increases dopamine levels and may help stop some of the withdrawal symptoms. Bupropion also tends to decrease the user's appetite.

As stated earlier, I have separated diet information on PCOS into a separate book titled, "The PCOS Diet," and in it you can read more on diet information if you are interested in it, but here I will very briefly cover some information on nutrients and nutrient timing known to be beneficial for those with

PCOS, before moving onto other health factors and a collection of ideas for cosmetic solutions.

CALORIES INTAKE TIMING

One study has indicated that the time of day when you ingest the most calories can have a significant effect on insulin and hormone levels. Lower insulin levels could help with fertility issues. The study, as reported by Michelle Konstantinovsky on One Medical, indicated that when women ate their largest portion of calories at breakfast, their glucose and insulin levels improved and they saw a fifty percent decrease in their testosterone levels. The recommended calorie count is approximately 980 for breakfast, 640 for lunch, and 190 for supper.

In addition to timing the number of calories you ingest, your doctor may recommend that you lower your calorie intake overall. Reducing your weight, even by five or ten pounds, can have a significant impact on your PCOS symptoms, including fertility issues.

Restrict Carbohydrates

Carbohydrates, such as sugars, increases insulin levels. Therefore, cutting foods that have a high carbohydrate content can help reduce symptoms of PCOS by helping you lose weight and decreasing blood sugars.

Keto Diet

The Keto diet restricts carbohydrate intake and focuses on increasing natural fats and proteins so that the body uses ketones to burn body fat. Ruled.Me, a website that provides resources for women with PCOS, recommends starting a Keto diet that consists of less than thirty-five grams of carbohydrates each day.

There are a lot of vegetables that can be eaten with the Keto diet. Of course, dark leafy greens are a great choice, as they have low carbs but have a lot of good nutrients. Broccoli, cauliflower, zucchini, and other similar vegetables are great for the Keto diet. Ruled.Me states that the more colorful and brighter the vegetable is, the fewer carbs it has.

Reducing the number of starchy vegetables is important, as the starches convert to carbs. These include potatoes, yams, peas, corn, and quinoa. Sweeter vegetables, like carrots, tend to have more carbs.

Many recipes for Keto-friendly dishes can be found on the internet. Check out the following websites to get started:

1. https://www.delish.com/cooking/g4798/easy-keto-diet-dinner-recipes/
2. https://www.allrecipes.com/recipes/22959/healthy-recipes/keto-diet/
3. https://www.dietdoctor.com/low-carb/keto/recipes
4. https://theinspiredhome.com/articles/31-tasty-keto-recipes-for-dinner-and-dessert

Fiber

Fiber is an important part of every diet. Foods that have a high fiber content can be especially important because they reduce inflammation and can reduce insulin resistance.

Reduce AGEs

Advanced glycation end products (AGEs) form when glucose and protein bind together. They have been connected to aging and degenerative diseases. One study suggests that cutting down on AGEs will decrease insulin levels, which in turn, can help with fertility. Processed foods and meat that has been cooked with high heat are high in AGEs. Cooking foods at a lower heat with moisture can reduce AGEs. Stewing, poaching, boiling, and steaming foods are a better option over searing or grilling.

Increase Vitamin D and Calcium

Vitamin D and calcium can help improve the symptoms of PCOS. In one study, infertile women with PCOS who consumed a thousand milligrams of calcium daily, a hundred thousand international units of vitamin D over six months, and fifteen hundred milligrams of metformin experienced improvements in their menstrual cycles, BMI, and other symptoms associated with PCOS.

Foods that are high in vitamin D include salmon, sardines, herring, cod liver oil, tuna, oysters, shrimp, egg yolks, mushrooms, and fortified foods (such as vitamin D cow milk, soy milk, orange juice, cereal, and oatmeal).

Calcium-rich foods include dairy products, seeds, sardines, salmon, some leafy greens (spinach, kale, and collards), legumes, beans, almonds, fortified foods and drinks, tofu, and edamame.

Magnesium

Magnesium is another supplement that might help you with your symptoms of PCOS because it may lower your insulin resistance.

Dark chocolate is a great source of magnesium and manganese, and it has prebiotic fibers that help feed the healthy bacteria in your gut. Dark chocolate also has antioxidants that help lower bad cholesterol.

Avocados are high in magnesium, fiber, and good fat.

Nuts are high in magnesium, fiber, and good fat. Studies indicate that nuts can improve blood sugar and cholesterol for people who suffer from type 2 diabetes. Legumes, tofu, seeds, whole grains, leafy greens, bananas, whole grains, and fatty fish also are high in magnesium, fiber, and other important nutrients.

Chromium

Chromium has been shown to decrease blood sugar levels and insulin resistance. One study showed that taking two hundred milligrams of chromium each day had the same effect on reducing insulin resistance as taking Metformin.

Chromium is found in a lot of food, including vegetables, whole grains, fruit, meat, and dairy products.

Web MD states that it is important to note that chromium can interfere with thyroid medication, so if you take thyroid medication, it is essential that you talk with your doctor before adding any kind of chromium supplements or adding a lot of chromium-rich foods to your diet.

Omega 3

Omega-3 fatty acids have demonstrated an ability to lower testosterone and to help women resume normal menstrual cycles. As noted in chapter two, sardines, herring, wild salmon, and farmed oysters are good sources of omega-3 fatty acids. Canola oil and soybean oil also have fatty acids in them. Walnuts, tofu, and leafy green vegetables are also a good source of omega-3 fatty acids. You can also take fish oil supplements, either by themselves or with vitamin D, which can increase your levels of fatty acids.

Nutritional Supplements

When people hear the word "supplement," they tend to think of bottles of pills found at the grocery store or health stores. However, supplements are also foods that you can add to your daily diet. There are several natural, nutritional supplements that you can use to reduce or even reverse the symptoms of PCOS.

1. Flax seeds have been shown to decrease androgen levels and insulin levels. Eating about a tablespoon and a half of flax seeds every day can also help you lose weight and inches from your waist. They can be added to salads, put in smoothies, or turned into a seed butter snack.

2. Cinnamon can reduce insulin resistance and increase ovarian function. Even a half to a full teaspoon of cinnamon each day can have a positive effect on your health.

3. Nuts, especially walnuts and almonds, can increase the hormone-binding globulin and decrease levels of androgens produced.

4. Studies indicate that berberine, found in foods such as Oregon grape root, goldenseal, and barberry, lowers insulin resistance as much as Metformin. It also contributes to greater fat and weight reduction. According to Ruled.Me, five hundred milligrams of berberine should be taken two or three times each day. Coconut oil and milk thistle can help your body

digest the berberine.

5. Apple cider vinegar also helps reduce insulin
    resistance. One study showed that after taking one
    tablespoon of vinegar daily, four of seven women
    began ovulating, six women had a significant
    reduction in insulin resistance, and five women
    decreased the number of androgens they produced.
    Apple cider vinegar can be used in cooking, sauces,
    and on salads.

6. Zinc is an element that aids in the function of
    hormones, enzymes, and immunity. In studies, zinc
    has shown to decrease the growth of body hair. The
    recommended dosage is two hundred twenty
    milligrams of zinc sulfate daily. This is great news if
    you love dark chocolate because dark chocolate is a
    source of zinc. Unfortunately, it is also a high-calorie
    food. Other foods that are rich in zinc include meat,
    shellfish, legumes, seeds, nuts, dairy foods, eggs, and
    whole grains.

7. Studies indicate that adding inositol in your diet can
    increase your menstrual cycles, improve insulin
    resistance, and decrease the production of male
    hormones. Food that contains inositol are eggs, meat,
    whole grains, legumes, sprouts, nuts, seeds, and many
    vegetables. According to Ruled.Me, taking between
    twelve hundred and twenty-four hundred milligrams
    of inositol daily can help significantly reduce
    symptoms of PCOS.

8. Vitamin B-9, also known as folic acid, is an essential
    addition for women who wish to become pregnant.

Ruled.Me states that women at a normal weight should take four hundred micrograms of folic acid daily, while overweight and obese women should take five milligrams daily. Kale, cabbage, broccoli, cauliflower, and asparagus are good sources of folic acid.

9. According to one study, walnuts may benefit women who have been diagnosed with PCOS. One woman stated that after she added walnuts to her diet, she began to have regular periods, which was something she had never experienced before. Her facial hair growth also decreased.

Moderate Exercise

Health experts suggest that women who suffer from PCOS should participate in at least thirty minutes of low to moderate exercises daily. It can help you decrease your weight and insulin resistance. This can increase your fertility and help you achieve regular menstrual cycles. It can also help reduce the male hormones your body produces, which in turn, can help reduce the baldness, facial hair, and acne.

In one study, women with PCOS participated in resistance training three times a week for four weeks, and as a result, lost weight and decreased the levels of androgens they produced.

Another study showed that fifty-six percent of women who did not menstruate began menstruating after doing aerobic exercises for twelve weeks.

One thing to keep in mind is not to overdo it. Too much exercise or losing too much weight can also disrupt your hormone balance as well. Healthline recommends yoga and pilates, but as with every treatment, you should talk to your doctor before getting started.

Stress

Stress is a part of life, but reducing stress levels in your life can help your PCOS symptoms improve. Here are a few ways to lower your stress levels:

1. Exercise is the number one way to reduce stress according to Healthline. Exercising decreases your stress hormones. It also helps you sleep, which is essential to reducing stress and improving your emotional well-being. Exercising can also promote confidence, which also reduces stress.

2. Supplements such as green tea, omega 3s, and lemon balm have been proven to lower stress.

3. Essential oils are known to reduce anxiety and stress, especially lavender, sandalwood, orange, and geranium, among others.

4. Caffeine can increase anxiety. Therefore, one way to decrease anxiety and stress is to decrease the amount of caffeine you ingest every day. Caffeine is not only in your coffee and sodas but can also be found in tea, chocolate, and other foods.

5. Keep a journal. Many people find that writing down their stresses and worries helps them deal with their worries more effectively. Conversely, writing down everything you are grateful for in your life can help you focus on the positive aspects of life instead of the issues that are stressing you out.

6. Studies indicate that chewing gum can help reduce

stress. It is thought that chewing gum promotes blood flow to the brain. Another thought is that chewing gum creates the same brain waves that are found in people who are relaxed.

7. Social support is another important way to relieve stress. According to Healthline, being a part of a social group gives you a sense of well-being and increases your self-esteem. Hanging out with friends and family increases the amount of oxytocin released in your brain, which is a hormone that releases stress and creates a feeling of well-being. Oxytocin creates the opposite effect of fight or flight.

8. Laughter truly is the best medicine. Not only does it help decrease stress and relieve muscle tension, but it can also increase your natural immunity.

9. One difficult way to relieve stress is to learn to say "no." This is especially true if you tend to take on more activities or jobs than you can handle that leave you feeling overwhelmed.

10. Avoiding procrastination may reduce stress. First, you have the items on your to-do list weighing heavily on your mind. Second, you are left scrambling at the last minute trying to get everything accomplished. To manage this habit, create a to-do list based on priorities and include reasonable deadlines. Then work your way down the list. Schedule specific times to accomplish specific tasks.

11. Practice mindfulness, which is focusing on the present moment. Acknowledge your negative thoughts and then bring your attention back to the

here and now. Studies show that mindfulness can increase self-esteem, which reduces stress, anxiety, and depression

12. Cuddling, hugging, and other physical contact increases oxytocin and decreases cortisol, a hormone produced by the adrenal glands.

13. Music has been proven to relieve stress. Soft, soothing music lowers your blood pressure, lowers your heart rate, and lowers your stress hormones. Listening to nature sounds can have a similar effect.

14. Breathing exercises, as discussed in chapter two, can help reduce stress. These exercises help you focus on your breathing technique and not on the negative thoughts that are causing you stress or anxiety.

15. Pets have been shown to greatly reduce stress. Spending time with your pet can trigger your brain to release oxytocin. Also, according to Healthline, pets help keep you active, give you a purpose, and provide you with companionship, all of which reduces stress and anxiety.

Sleep

Getting a good night's sleep allows your body the opportunity to rejuvenate itself and alleviates stress and anxiety. However, research indicates that women who suffer from PCOS are twice as likely to suffer from interrupted sleep or insomnia than other women. In chapter two there are several suggestions that can help you improve your sleep.

Meditation

Meditation is a very popular method used to decrease stress and anxiety levels. It lowers cortisol levels and insulin resistance. Meditating a half-hour before you go to bed can help improve your sleep while reducing the effect of stressful thoughts.

Medication

Doctors may prescribe a birth control pill or a combination of birth control pills that can increase estrogen and progestin while decreasing androgens. Some of these birth control medications can help slow balding and hair growth as well.

If you are trying to get pregnant, the doctor may prescribe progestin therapy, which can help protect you from endometrial cancer.

There are also medications the doctors can prescribe to help you ovulate if you are trying to get pregnant. In addition, Metformin may be prescribed to lower insulin resistance and insulin levels. Not only can this increase your fertility, but it can also help prevent prediabetes from developing into type 2 diabetes.

Cosmetic Solutions

Acne

Contrary to popular belief, acne is not a problem that only affects teenagers. Women who suffer from PCOS often suffer from acne. However, Kristeen Cherney has written an article on Healthline that describes several ways you can deal with this issue.

Because this acne is caused by an excess of androgens, birth control or anti-androgen drugs that reduce the levels of male hormones you produce can be prescribed for you.

Some people blame excessive acne on food and say that junk food, such as chocolate and French fries, can cause acne.

However, Cherney states that there is no evidence of a direct link. However, some foods can cause increased inflammation in the body. Red meat, white potatoes, white bread, and sugary desserts are a few examples of such foods. On the flip side of this, there are a lot of foods that can decrease inflammation such as walnuts, tomatoes, spinach, kale, almonds, olive oil, berries, salmon, and turmeric.

Anti-inflammatory supplements like zinc, vitamins A & C, garlic, copper, and bromelain can also be beneficial.

Cherney recommends washing your face twice daily to reduce oil build-up. After washing your face, you should use an oil-free moisturizer. You should also only use noncomedogenic makeup. Resist the temptation to pop, pick, or scratch at pimples that pop up as this can cause scarring.

Excessive Hair

More and more women are embracing their facial and other body hair as just another part of who they are.

Harnaam Kaur was diagnosed with PCOS when she was twelve. After trying several remedies, such as waxing and shaving, she decided that she would let her hair grow out at the age of sixteen. She was able to grow a full beard. Today, she is a model and a body confidence advocate. Harnaam has some great advice for any woman who struggles with PCOS: "One in five women have polycystic ovaries and lots of them approach me about how to counter the bullying and how to accept themselves. I want them to say: 'Well, Harnaam is on the catwalk, why not me?' Bearded ladies were once laughed at – I want to break the mold."

She is not the only woman who is embracing and loving herself regardless of whether or not she has facial hair. Alma

Torres noticed that she had facial and neck hair when she was around nine or ten years old. It continued to grow, and she remembers having to shave her thick, dark sideburns for her eighth-grade prom. She began to shave her face daily until one day she stopped. Alma says she is glad she stopped shaving because her beard has boosted her confidence. She tells *Allure Magazine*, "I fell in love with what I couldn't change about myself. I love myself a little more than I did before, and it's OK to be different from everyone else. We were born to stand out. Change for no one but yourself."

There are many other women who share the sentiments of Alma and Harnaam. Annalisa Hackleman decided to walk a similar path of self-love. After years of doing everything—shaving four times a day, threading, waxing, laser treatments—with no solution, she was having meltdowns. Her husband encouraged her to just give her face a rest. Now she embraces her beard and who she is. She tells *Allure,* "The biggest thing I want people to take away from my story is that you can empower yourself—you don't have to be a slave to something you hate. If you hate the hair, remove it, or flip it and learn to love it. Whatever you choose to do, remember that other people can't decide what's right for you. You don't need anyone's approval for your body."

These three women, and many others who suffer from PCOS and excessive hair growth, offer the same message: Be true to yourself. Do not worry about what everyone else is thinking or saying. Do what is best for you and you alone.

If you are not quite ready to let your hair grow out, there are some other solutions that you can use to deal with the excessive hair growth caused by PCOS.

Waxing

According to registered nurse, Nicole Galan, waxing is the most preferred method of hair removal by women who suffer from PCOS, especially when dealing with that pesky facial hair. Galan says that most women like it because it is easy and affordable. However, there are some side effects to waxing.

1. The pain resulting from waxing may vary, depending on the person. Galan states that one way you can help reduce the discomfort is to take Tylenol or Advil about an hour before you start. Then, you can try icing the area after the treatment.

Galan recommends trimming or shaving longer hairs before waxing to help the wax grab the hairs more easily. She also recommends doing your research and getting references to ensure you're going to a salon that has the skills and experience to minimize the pain. There are ever waxers who specialize in working with women who have PCOS.

1. If you have sensitive skin or if it is your first few times waxing, you may get red bumps forming on your skin. Galan states that the bumps usually only last one or two days and will lessen with each waxing.

Gently exfoliating to get rid of debris and dirt may help prevent the red bumps from appearing. Applying a warm compress to the area that is to be waxed may also help, as it opens up your pores. This helps the hairs come out easier and makes the waxing less painful. Using hydrocortisone cream can soothe the irritation.

1. Infections are not a normal side effect of waxing. However, they can occur if the salon does not change out the wax between clients. It is important that you see a doctor if you experience swelling, warmth, itching, or pain. You might have to use an anti-bacterial cream or take an oral antibiotic.

2. Skin discoloration might occur if the waxed areas are exposed to the sun soon after the waxing. You might be especially prone to the sun's effects if you are taking birth control pills or some antibiotics. It is important that you always use sunscreen on the waxed areas. If you do experience discoloration, you can cover it with concealer or other makeup. You might also consider a different choice of hair removal if the issue continues.

3. You might experience ingrown hairs after waxing. Galan says that ingrown hairs occur when the hair is torn or cut instead of removed. The hair then coils into the skin. Exfoliating before waxing can help prevent ingrown hairs since it removes dead skin and keeps the hair pointing in the right direction.

4. Torn, ripped, and bruised skin is another potential side effect of waxing. People who are taking certain medications, including hormone replacements and birth control, may have extra sensitive skin and should check with their doctor before getting waxed.

Electrolysis

Electrolysis is another way that women with PCOS choose to get rid of body hair, especially facial hair. Women may choose this method because it is a permanent way to get rid of unwanted hair. It is the only FDA approved method for permanently removing hair.

With this remedy, the technician will insert a needle into the hair follicle, then apply a small amount of electricity to kill the follicle. Tweezers are used to remove the hair. Because your hair grows in three phases, you will need multiple treatments.

Before you head off to visit the aesthetician, you should avoid sunlight for a minimum of two to three days before your appointment. You should also not pluck or wax your hair for as long as possible prior to your appointment. In addition, you should avoid taking caffeine or alcohol before your visit.

After your appointment, you should avoid sunlight for a couple of days. Your aesthetician may also advise you to not wash your face or use makeup for a specific length of time after your treatment. You may also receive an antibiotic or hydrocortisone cream to use on the area to help prevent infection.

However, there are some considerations you should think about before heading to the technician's office.

1. Galan says that because everyone's pain tolerance is different, electrolysis can be painful for some and only mildly annoying for others. The discomfort comes from having the needle inserted into the follicles repeatedly, which Galan describes as a slight stinging feeling.

You can take some Tylenol or Advil before your appointment to help with the discomfort. There are some topical creams and sprays that can be used to numb the skin before the process, although you should check with your aesthetician before applying them.

1. Electrolysis can be expensive, costing anywhere from several hundred dollars to more than a thousand dollars. However, treatments are spread out over time, and many practitioners have a "pay as you go" policy.
2. Make sure that you choose an aesthetician who is licensed to perform electrolysis. Also, make sure to check the technician's references.

Laser Removal

Another way of removing facial hair is through laser removal, although it has not been approved by the FDA. This method involves a hot, intense light beam that is focused on the hair follicles to destroy them. Like electrolysis, this technique can take several sessions.

It is very important to make sure that the aesthetician who is performing your laser hair removal is licensed and experienced. Make sure that you check references and testimonials of former clients before committing to a technician.

Similar to waxing and electrolysis, there are important issues you should consider before getting this treatment.

1. Even though it is widely considered to be a

permanent solution for dealing with facial hair, some women with PCOS have found it to be totally ineffective. Annalisa Hackleman, who now sports a full bread, reported that the laser treatments did not work at all for her.

2. Each woman's pain tolerance is different. Galan says that most people describe the feeling as being similar to having a rubber band snapped against the skin repeatedly.

The positive side to this is that laser treatment sessions are short and can be completed very quickly, so most women find the discomfort tolerable. You can also take painkillers like Tylenol or Advil about an hour before your treatment to minimize the pain. The technician may also allow you to apply a topical anesthetic prior to treatment.

1. Laser treatments can be costly. Luckily, since multiple sessions are necessary to see results, most clinics allow you to pay as you go.

Tweezing/Plucking

Plucking and tweezing are methods that are best used on smaller areas with less hair. The pain is minimal, and most people don't experience any discomfort at all. However, removing hair strand by strand can be a bit monotonous, time-consuming, and annoying.

Threading

Threading is an ancient technique used by Indian and central Asian women. Regular sewing thread is wrapped around several hairs at once and then tugged to remove the hair. Like any process where the hair is pulled out of the follicles, it can be uncomfortable. However, most women say that it is not as bad as waxing. Witch Hazel can soothe any redness, itching, and pain after this procedure.

Shaving

Shaving is the old standby for a lot of women and causes the least amount of pain of all the hair removal techniques. However, you have to shave often because the blade simply cuts the hair off at the skin level, as opposed to completely removing it.

Use new razors with sharp blades to avoid cutting yourself. Shaving cream can help prevent irritation and red bumps, as can moisturizers.

Sugaring

Some women use a method called sugaring to get rid of their unwanted facial hair. The idea behind sugaring is very similar to waxing. A sugar solution can be made from items commonly found in your food pantry, such as sugar, vinegar, lime juice, honey, etc.

Sugaring can be uncomfortable since pulling hair out of your face is never fun. Compared to waxing, though, it may be a little easier to bear because it is less likely to tear or rip your skin. However, some women say it can be more uncomfortable than waxing, depending on the temperature of the sugar solution.

Medications

There are some medications that you can take that might be able to help you with excessive hair growth. Galan states that two of these medications, Vaniqa and Flutamide, are designed to help correct the hormonal imbalances that cause excessive hair growth. Some of these medications are oral, while others come in the form of a cream you can apply to the afflicted area.

Depilatories

There are creams and lotions that are designed for removing hair. Galan says most of these products, although pungent, are not painful. However, some women have reported feeling a slight stinging or burning sensation after application.

If you use one of these creams, and you experience pain, you should wash it off immediately. If the pain does not go away quickly, then you should call a doctor. Galan says that pain can be a sign of having a bad reaction to one of the ingredients in the product.

Another potential negative issue with chemical depilatories is that they can cause chemical burns on your face. It is very important that you follow the directions explicitly when you are using these types of products.

Thinning or Baldness

PCOS can cause thinning hair or male pattern baldness. Longhurst writes in her Healthline article that the hair you lose due to PCOS will not grow back by itself. However, there are ways to promote new hair growth, or to deal with thinning hair and bald patches.

Hormone Therapy

Hormone therapy may help stop hair loss and may even promote new hair growth. The hormone therapy balances out your hormone production and reduces the androgens produced by your body. This is usually delivered in the form of birth control.

Rogaine

Rogaine is the only over the counter medication that can be used to treat thinning hair. It is applied directly to the thinning areas. One problem with Rogaine is that once you stop using it, your hair will start to thin again.

Other Medications

There are other medications doctors may prescribe to help decrease testosterone levels. Galan emphasizes that there have not been a lot of scientific studies regarding the use of these medications to treat thinning hair and hair loss.

1. Spironolactone is a diuretic but is also used to treat hair loss. It is often prescribed along with birth control. It can be used at the same time you are using Rogaine.

2. Finasteride is a medication that is normally prescribed to men to prevent prostate growth. This medication helps treat baldness and thinning hair by preventing the testosterone from binding with your hair follicles. It is essential that birth control is used at the same time because this medication can have a negative effect on your pregnancy.

3. Flutamide also prevents the testosterone from binding with hair follicles. It cannot be taken while you are pregnant or breastfeeding. As a matter of fact,

Galan warns that this medication is not used very often in the United States because it is so toxic.

Hair Transplant

Some women opt for a medical procedure where hair and hair follicles are removed from one area of the body that has a lot of hair and transplanted to the areas of the scalp where the hair is thinning. This usually requires several procedures to be completed. Unfortunately, the transplants are not always successful, even after several procedures.

The other problem with this procedure is that it can be cost-prohibitive. Hair transplants can cost up to fifteen thousand dollars in some cases.

Zinc

Longhurst states that there are studies that indicate zinc may help with thinning and baldness. One study showed that taking fifty milligrams of elemental zinc each day for eight weeks had a positive effect on participants. The same study also showed that taking zinc supplements helped reduce excessive hair growth.

Biotin

Biotin is another supplement that people use to try to treat thinning hair. Longhurst states that there are no studies that show that biotin is effective for women suffering from PCOS. However, she does say that one study completed in 2015 showed that biotin taken in a marine supplement did help some women PCOS, although exact statistics were not provided.

Making It Less Obvious

There are ways that you can make your thinning hair and androgen pattern baldness less noticeable. If your part is widening, you might consider parting your hair in a different place. Longhurst suggests getting bangs that begin farther up on the scalp as one option. Another option is using root cover-up powder, which is waterproof and comes in a variety of colors and shades.

A partial wig, or wig fall, can cover the parts of your head where you are experiencing thinning. These can be worn without clips or glue that can damage your hair. Volumizing products can be used to make your hair look fuller. A short hairstyle, with layered hair, can also help add volume and fullness.

Bald patches can also be masked. Longhurst suggests using a ponytail or top not to hold the hair in place over the bald spots. You can also use a hairband or scarf to cover the bald spots.

Bottom Line

You have to feel comfortable with yourself. As Annalisa Hackleman said, you have to do what is right for you. You do not have to have anyone else's approval about you or your body.

Reducing Symptoms of PCOS

There are a lot of ways to reduce the symptoms of PCOS. Some solutions are more effective than others. However, there are many studies that show that a diagnosis of PCOS is not a diagnosis of doom. It is treatable.

Chapter Summary

- There are many ways to reverse and reduce the symptoms of PCOS.

- Lifestyle changes, including exercise, diet, and sleep can reduce insulin resistance and resist the number of androgens produced by the body.

- Lifestyle changes and medications can help increase fertility for women suffering from PCOS.

In the next chapter, you will learn about insulin's relationship with PCOS.

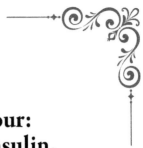

Chapter Four:
PCOS and Insulin,
What's the Relation?

Think of insulin the way you would a chocolate cake. You have to get just enough of it to be satisfied. If you get too small a slice, then your whole body is left wanting more, and that is all you can think about—just a little bit more, please. If you get too big a slice and eat it, then you get sick. Your stomach hurts, your head hurts, and you just want to curl up in a ball and be left alone. You get the perfect amount, and all's right with the world.

Unfortunately, while the effects of chocolate cake are short-term, the effects of getting too much or too little insulin are not.

Insulin's job is to break down the food you eat, like that yummy chocolate cake or an amazing steak dinner, into simple sugars or glucose, so that it can be used as energy. Insulin moves the sugars into the different cells in the body, so the cells have energy. It also encourages your liver and muscles to absorb the glucose.

Insulin, a hormone produced in the pancreas, increases right after you eat, does it's job, and then decreases. However, if your body does not produce enough insulin then you end up with high blood sugar. When your body does not use insulin properly, such as in the case of insulin resistance, a whole host of new problems surface, such as PCOS and type 2 diabetes.

Insulin resistance occurs when your body has to have higher than normal levels of insulin to deal with the glucose levels. Then, even after the glucose levels return to normal, the insulin levels are high, indicating that the pancreas had to create higher than normal amounts of insulin to process the sugars. There are different causes of insulin resistance, including being overweight and genetics.

According to Dr. Lara Briden, most women with PCOS are resistant to insulin or have high insulin levels. She states that insulin resistance is not only a symptom of PCOS and a contributor to PCOS. One of the ways to diagnose PCOS is to measure the amount of insulin in the blood.

Dr. Briden points out that while PCOS does affect the ovaries, it is not a disease of just the ovaries. In fact, it is a disease that affects the entire endocrine system and metabolic system and is related to insulin resistance.

Effects of Insulin Resistance

Studies indicate that insulin resistance contributes to PCOS. According to Dr. Briden, seventy to ninety-five percent of obese women who suffer from PCOS are also insulin resistant. Thirty to seventy-five percent of lean women who suffer from PCOS are also insulin resistant.

Insulin resistance can weaken ovulation, which in turn, decreases fertility. It also decreases the menstrual cycles, resulting in a build-up of the endometrial fluid in the uterus. This can cause endometrial cancer.

There are several symptoms caused by insulin resistance. One symptom is thick, dark patches of skin on the neck, under your arms, and in your groin area. The insulin resistance can cause the ovaries to produce excessive androgens, such as testosterone, in women who suffer from PCOS. The extra production of androgens can result in excessive acne, excessive hair growth on the face, chest, and other body areas, as well as thinning hair and male pattern baldness.

In addition, insulin resistance can lead to type 2 diabetes and weight gain.

Decreasing Insulin Resistance

The good news is that there are ways to deal with insulin resistance. Insulin resistance and blood sugar levels can be decreased, which in turn, can decrease the symptoms of PCOS.

Diet is one important tool you can use to control your insulin levels. Eating foods that are lower in starches and sugars, yet are higher in fiber, can naturally lower your blood sugar and insulin levels. In addition, you should avoid foods that have a high amount of refined carbohydrates.

The amount of fructose you consume can make a difference in your insulin sensitivity. Lower amounts of fructose, as is found in fruit, can actually improve insulin sensitivity. However, higher amounts of fructose from sodas, fruit juices, and desserts can hurt insulin sensitivity.

Exercise is another way to reduce the insulin and blood sugar levels. As mentioned, any amount of exercise can help reduce insulin levels and improve PCOS symptoms, although a minimum of thirty to sixty minutes of exercise per day is recommended by Healthline. Dr. Briden recommends aerobic exercises and resistance training.

Medication is also used to control insulin levels. Metformin, one of the main medications used to control the glucose in the blood, makes you more sensitive to insulin and decreases the amount of glucose released by your liver. Studies have shown that Metformin, combined with a healthy diet and exercise, helps reduce the risk of developing type 2 diabetes. In addition, it helps women who have PCOS lose weight and keep it off. Metformin also helps lower cholesterol.

Supplements

Supplements can be taken either in pill or powder form from a bottle or via food products. While the bottle form can be convenient and ensures you are getting a specific amount, there are many food products that provide several of the different vitamins and minerals that you need all at once.

There are many supplements that can help increase insulin sensitivity. Many of these supplements were discussed in chapter three, as they also help treat or reverse many symptoms of PCOS. These supplements include inositol, chromium, cinnamon, zinc, berberine, and a combination of vitamin D and calcium. There are additional supplements that you can add to your diet as well.

1. Cod liver oil has vitamins A and D, and omega 3 fatty acids. Taking this supplement can help regulate your menstrual cycle and reduce fat around your waist.

2. Evening primrose oil can help reduce the pain associated with menstruation and can also help regulate menstrual cycles.

3. Turmeric is another supplement that may be able to

decrease insulin resistance, and to reduce inflammation.

Reducing Androgen Levels

While reducing insulin resistance can help decrease the androgen levels created by the ovaries, there are other supplements that can also balance the levels of the male hormones in the body.

1. Maca root has been used to increase fertility. It also may be used to decrease cortisol and balance hormone levels. In addition, maca root may help reduce depression.
2. Indian root, otherwise known as ashwagandha, can help balance the levels of cortisol, which helps reduce stress and depression and also can help improve the symptoms of PCOS.
3. Holy basil, or tulsi, reduces cortisol and blood sugar levels and helps prevent weight gain.
4. Licorice root can help reduce inflammation. It may also be able to balance hormones and metabolize sugar.

Probiotics

Probiotics are live bacteria and yeast. Considered to be "good" bacteria, they help keep your gut healthy. They are found in a lot of food such as yogurt, kefir, sauerkraut, kimchi, miso, pickles, and buttermilk.

One study, reported by the American Diabetes Association, found that taking probiotics can have a significant impact on PCOS symptoms. Researchers tested seventy-eight women with PCOS. The researchers treated some of the women with Metformin and some of the women with probiotics for three weeks. Both groups of women improved their menstrual cycles, and they experienced a decrease in insulin resistance and the production of androgens.

Therefore, by targeting the bacteria in the gut, women with PCOS were able to treat their symptoms by increasing probiotics in their diet.

Chapter Summary

- Insulin resistance is a significant contributor to PCOS.

- Insulin resistance causes the ovaries to produce male hormones, which causes excessive hair growth, male pattern baldness, and excessive acne.

- Insulin resistance contributes to infertility.

- There are many natural foods and supplements you can take that can help decrease your insulin resistance and help reverse many of the symptoms of PCOS.

- One study indicated that probiotics and Metformin may produce similar results when treating insulin resistance.

In the next chapter, you will learn about whether birth control can help with fertility issues and reduce or reverse PCOS symptoms.

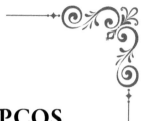

Chapter Five: PCOS and Hormones

The consortium that was mentioned in chapter one recommended that birth control pills be the first drug used to assist with regulating your menstrual cycle and help control the levels of male and female hormones.

It is very important to work with your doctor to find the right solution for you. Going back to Lusinski's article, we encounter a woman with PCOS named Andrea who experienced heavy bleeding for three months straight. When she told her doctor about the bleeding, her concerns were dismissed and she was told heavy bleeding was a typical symptom of PCOS. She then went to the emergency room where she was informed that she had lost so much blood that she was almost at the point of needing a transfusion. Sadly, Andrea's struggles with misinformed doctors did not end there. She told another doctor that she did not like the birth control she was on because it made her depressed, suicidal, and anxious. She was told that she would either have to continue taking the birth control pill she was on or bleed until her body decided to stop bleeding. Of course, neither of these options were helpful to Andrea. Once again, she was dealing with a doctor who hadn't considered all of the other options available for women with PCOS. After much searching, Andrea was finally able to get on a birth control pill that not only controls her bleeding but also does not cause anxiety, depression, and suicidal thoughts. Had her original doctor been more informed about treatment options for PCOS, she would have been spared this struggle.

Combination Birth Control

Women with PCOS are often prescribed combination birth control, which is birth control that has two hormones: Estrogen and progesterone. The purpose of combination birth control is to increase the levels of estrogen your ovaries produce while reducing the amount of androgens produced.

Combination birth control is often used because it treats many PCOS-related symptoms. Women who take combination birth control may begin to ovulate more regularly. This leads to lighter periods and more regular periods. Because the endometrial lining of the uterus is shed more often, women tend to have fewer cramps and also have a lower chance of developing endometrial cancer and ovarian cysts. Because the combination birth control lowers the amount of androgens produced, you will likely have clearer skin, less facial hair, and less balding and thinning of the hair.

Risks of Combination Birth Control and Hormone Treatments

According to Zawn Villines, writing for Medical News Today, while most women can safely take birth control pills, there are some risks.

Birth control can cause problems with insulin resistance. This means birth control pills create a higher risk for diabetes. This can be a significant problem since women with PCOS are already at a higher risk for diabetes.

Another health risk for women with PCOS is that hormonal birth control pills can create an increased risk for cardiovascular problems, including blood clots that form in the legs. Women with PCOS, especially women who are overweight or obese, are already at a greater risk. Smoking increases this risk even more.

Some studies indicate that hormonal birth control can cause weight gain, although more research is needed to confirm this claim. Some women who are already overweight or obese may be reluctant to take hormonal birth control because they fear additional weight gain.

Women who take combination birth control to treat their PCOS may face additional side effects. They may suffer from mood changes, sore breasts, headaches, nausea, and spotting. Some women also suffer from weight loss.

Other Options

There are other hormonal treatments for women with PCOS besides combination birth control.

1. Minipills are progestin-only pills. The increased progestin can help regulate menstrual periods and lower your risk for endometrial cancer.
2. Skin patches, which contain estrogen and progestin, can be worn for twenty one days. It is taken off for seven days, and a new one is put on. The effects are the same as taking a daily oral combination pill. Users may also experience skin irritation and high blood pressure.
3. A vaginal ring is another option. It is inserted into the vagina for twenty one days and then taken out for

seven days during the menstrual cycle. A new one is inserted after the cycle. The ring can help you ovulate, regulate your menstrual cycle and reduce bloating, cramps, the risk of endometrial cancer, and excessive body hair growth. The negative effects are the same as the oral combination pills, with the additional potential side effects of dizziness and fatigue.

4. A Mirena intrauterine device (IUD) is another option for women who are not trying to get pregnant. It releases progestin. While many women find their PCOS symptoms disappear after using the device without issue, some experience chronic abdominal pain. This is just another example of how treatments affect women differently.

Metformin

Metformin is a drug that is used to treat diabetes and insulin resistance. However, many doctors prescribe Metformin as a way to help women maintain their hormone balance. The reason? Excessive androgen production can contribute to insulin resistance.

The results for this treatment are varied as well. Some women claim that their symptoms have improved. However, there are others who report that the drug simply made them feel dizzy and nauseous.

Diet

Diet can play a big part in the hormones your body produces. Dea, a Clue Ambassador (an advocate for women with PCOS), stated that she had told her doctors that she did not want to use pills or any other kind of medications that would use hormones to regulate her periods. Instead, she chose to balance her hormones through her diet. Dea carefully researched different foods to see which foods would cause a hormone imbalance. While Dea said that she cannot say for sure her diet is what contributed to her recovery, she no longer suffers from any of the symptoms of PCOS except for some ovarian cysts.

So, what foods can cause a hormonal imbalance? It probably won't surprise you to learn that most of these foods, if not all, are junk foods.

1. High fructose corn syrup will get you every time. Instead of eating high fructose corn syrup, try sweetening your food with maple, molasses, and regular corn syrup.

2. Artificial sweeteners can also cause hormone imbalances. Not only that, but there are several studies that indicate that artificial sweeteners increase your appetite and increase your motivation to eat. Since sugar can also cause hormonal imbalances, Abbey Sharp, RD, recommends that you simply decrease the amount of sweetener you use in general.

3. It is best to decrease the amount of alcohol you consume, or eliminate it from your diet altogether.

4. There are studies that show a link between caffeine and estrogen changes, as well as changes in hormone behavior. Therefore, putting down that cup of "go juice" in the morning may bring you one step closer to balancing your hormones. Experts suggest drinking green tea if you must have that caffeine boost. Green tea has the added benefit of improving

insulin resistance.

There are several foods that you can eat that can help you regain and maintain a hormone balance.

1. Healthline suggests that soy products may help because they act like estrogen in your body. However, because soy products can interfere with your endocrine system, talk to your doctor before adding a lot of soy to your diet. This is especially necessary if there is a history of breast cancer or other estrogen-related cancers in your family.
2. Eating whole foods that have not been processed are a good way to help maintain a healthy hormonal balance as these foods have no hormones in them.
3. Adaptogen herbs, such as licorice root and chasteberry, can also be consumed to help balance hormonal irregularities. In addition, some of them may help with other symptoms of PCOS.

Probiotics can also help you maintain a healthy hormone balance by regulating androgens and estrogen.

What Do The Doctors Know?

Stories from women with PCOS of all ages prove one thing: Doctors do not know as much as they should regarding PCOS, and this includes information about how to balance the hormones that are causing some of your symptoms.

Many women, such as Dea, have said their doctors told them that the only way to balance their hormones was to go on birth control. In Dea's case, she rejected that advice and tried a naturalistic way to treat her PCOS and succeeded.

As we saw with Andrea and as many other women have experienced firsthand, doctors often jump to birth control as the only way to treat PCOS. This narrow approach to treatment can have huge consequences when doctors are unwilling to do further research. Doctors need to understand that one size does not fit all.

Chapter Summary

- As hormones are the key issue with PCOS, medications like birth control are the first treatment offered.

- Combination birth control containing estrogen and progestin are most commonly prescribed.

- Metformin may also be prescribed to help control hormone production.

- Some women have found changing their diets to be the only effective way to manage the hormonal imbalances they have suffered from.

In the next chapter, you will learn about PCOS, ovulation, and fertility.

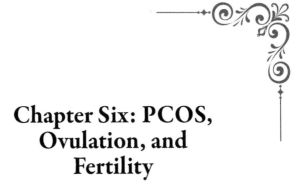

Chapter Six: PCOS, Ovulation, and Fertility

One of the most devastating symptoms of PCOS is infertility. Rebecca Andrews, who was diagnosed at age sixteen, actually had to have one of her ovaries removed because it was crushed by a cyst. She tried in-vitro fertilization, but unfortunately, suffered six miscarriages. She told ABC News that this was the worst aspect of PCOS for her. She also had to suffer through comments from ignorant people telling her to get used to it or get over it. No doubt, this is a story that will sound very familiar to any women with PCOS who has struggled with infertility.

While infertility is a symptom experienced by some women, a diagnosis of PCOS does not mean that you cannot have children. In fact, there are many ways that the symptoms of PCOS can be treated to increase the ability to conceive and give birth to healthy children.

In the article written by Lusinksi, Amy tells her story. She went to a doctor because she had missed many periods. The doctor simply gave her more birth control pills and told her it would be very difficult for her to get pregnant when she was ready for children and that she would have to "jump through hoops" to conceive, if she could at all. She now has three children.

Stephanie tells a similar story in Lusinksi's article. When she was diagnosed at the age of nineteen with PCOS, the doctor informed her that she had a "zero chance of getting pregnant without fertility treatments." Stephanie says that she was devastated when the doctor gave her this news. Fortunately, her doctor was wrong, and she became pregnant at the age of thirty-three on her and her husband's first try. Now, Stephanie wants all women like her to know that while PCOS can cause irregular menstrual cycles and can make it harder to get pregnant, it does not mean that women with PCOS cannot have children.

Hollie is another woman who was misinformed about her fertility. She was sixteen when she was diagnosed with PCOS and was told that she could never have children. When she was twenty-six, she visited a different doctor who told her the truth. She would be able to have children. Hollie was justifiably upset. She'd spent ten years depressed, devastated by the thought that she would never have children.

According to Jen Bell, a *Clue* writer who focuses on several topics, including PCOS, women with PCOS tend to need fertility treatments more than other women. However, Bell says the research shows that women with PCOS tend to have the same number of children over their lifetimes as women who do not have PCOS. Bell offers reassurance saying, "In fact, the majority of people with PCOS who are trying to conceive will become pregnant and give birth without any fertility treatment at least once in their life."

If you are one of the women who struggle to get pregnant, there are treatments that you and your doctor can try to improve your chances of becoming pregnant and safely carrying the baby to term.

On the flip side of this issue, you should use birth control if you are not ready for children. Although women with PCOS do not always ovulate on a regular, predictable basis, they may still ovulate.

It is important to remember that every woman experiences PCOS differently. This is true for fertility as well.

The Links Between PCOS and Infertility

There are three major possible links between PCOS and infertility. One potential cause of infertility is that it is more difficult for women who suffer from PCOS to ovulate. Ovulation can be hindered by the excessive amounts of testosterone in the body or the eggs may not mature.

Another possible cause is that the hormone imbalance may make it more difficult for the uterine lining to develop properly. That means that the egg is unable to be implanted.

Ovulation and menstruation are irregular and unpredictable. This can make it very difficult to figure out when you are fertile.

Weight Loss

Like every other potential solution with PCOS, one of the solutions recommended by doctors to increase fertility is to lose weight. However, this is easier said than done, especially for women with PCOS. It is difficult, but not impossible.

As noted earlier, even a weight loss of five to ten pounds is beneficial. A healthy diet coupled with performing aerobic exercises for thirty to sixty minutes a day can make a huge difference in your symptoms, including infertility.

Supplements

Supplements may also help increase fertility, although like everything else associated with PCOS, more research is needed. There is some evidence that black cohosh may help increase fertility. It can be used alone or in combination with Clomiphene.

Inositol is another supplement that may increase ovulation and help your menstrual cycles become regular. However, it can cause abdominal cramps or nausea.

Vitamin D supplements can help increase ovulation when you take it alone. When it is combined with Metformin, vitamin D can help you have more regulated menstrual cycles.

Medications

Your doctor may prescribe different medications to help you ovulate so that you can conceive. Some of the drugs may be prescribed alone or in combination with other medications.

1. Clomiphene and Letrozole are anti-estrogen medications that you would take at the beginning of your cycle. When the estrogen levels decrease, your pituitary gland produces more follicle-stimulating hormone (FSH). This means that the ovaries are encouraged to produce mature eggs in the egg sacs, so they can be released.

Letrozole is more effective when used alone, than Clomiphene is, according to Laurie Ray, a science writer at *Clue*.

One side effect of these two medications is that you may experience hot flashes. Ray explains that neither of these medications should be taken for more than six months.

1. Metformin seems to be the go-to medication for everything regarding PCOS, and it is no different when discussing fertility. Because PCOS and many of the resulting symptoms, including infertility, are caused by insulin resistance, Metformin is prescribed. When the levels of insulin decrease, this results in a better balance of hormone production.

Although Metformin does seem to have many of the answers regarding PCOS and its symptoms, Metformin does have side effects. Ray reports that some people who take Metformin experience diarrhea and abdominal pain. Other women have reported nausea as well.

Ray states that according to studies, fertility rates are increased when Metformin is used in conjunction with Clomiphene.

1. Fertility injections may be used if the oral medications are not effective. There are several medications available. These medications signal the ovaries to produce eggs.

These injections tend to cause several eggs to be released at once, resulting in a higher risk of having multiple births. You will need to have your blood checked regularly for estradiol levels, which is another hormone produced in the ovaries.

Timing

It is important that you time sex with your ovulation periods when you are trying to get pregnant. You need to track your menstrual cycle. You will likely be ovulating thirteen to fifteen days before your period starts.

Basal Body Temperature

One way to track your ovulation cycle is to take your temperature. Your resting temperature will rise slightly when you are ovulating. Take your temperature first thing in the morning before you sit up. Note that this method won't help you predict ovulation in the future.

Using a special basal body thermometer will provide a more accurate reading than a regular thermometer. You will need to take your temperature at the same time every day.

Ovulation Tests

There are ovulation tests that you can take at home. They are similar to pregnancy tests in that they measure the level of specific hormones in your body. The ovulation tests determine the amount of luteinizing hormone (LH) that is in your body, so you can figure out what your ovulation window is and when you will be fertile.

In-Vitro

In-vitro fertilization (IVF) has several steps. First, you would receive fertility injections every day. The injections cause the ovaries to produce several eggs. The eggs are harvested through a minor procedure. The doctor inserts a thin, hollow tube through your vagina and then into your ovaries and follicles to retrieve the mature eggs. According to Planned Parenthood, you will receive medication to help you stay comfortable during this procedure.

The eggs are then fertilized in a lab. They are monitored by the staff to make sure the cells are dividing into an embryo. A certain number of eggs are implanted into your uterus using a thin tube. Planned Parenthood states that this procedure is usually not painful.

If the eggs attach to the uterine wall, then pregnancy results. Because more than one fertilized embryo is often implanted, you may have multiple pregnancies.

After the egg or eggs are implanted, you will need to rest for a day after the transfer. Planned Parenthood says that it is safe to return to your normal activities the day after. In addition, you may take progesterone, either orally or through shots, for the first eight to ten weeks after the embryo is implanted. The progesterone helps the embryos survive in your uterus.

Any leftover fertilized eggs are cryopreserved, or frozen, for future pregnancies.

There are some potential side effects with IVF, just like there are for every other treatment associated with PCOS.

Planned Parenthood states that you might experience cramping, bloating, sore breasts, mood swings, headaches, bleeding, infections, bruising from the shots, and allergic reactions to the medication. Many people suffer from depression and anxiety while they are going through the IVF process.

Another potential issue with IVF is that it can be expensive. One cycle can cost fifteen thousand dollars or more. Some insurance plans cover IVF, but not all of them do. You might have to go through more than one cycle for a pregnancy to take.

Intrauterine Insemination

Intrauterine Insemination (IUI) is also known as artificial insemination. The doctor will place the sperm cells directly into your uterus when you are ovulating, which helps the sperm get closer to the egg. Before the procedure, semen is collected from your partner and washed. This means that a concentrated amount of healthy sperm is collected. If the sperm fertilizes your egg, and the egg attaches to your uterine wall, then you become pregnant.

Before the procedure, you will receive medications to help you develop mature eggs. Then, you will be given medication that makes you ovulate. The doctor will figure out when the egg is ready and waiting to be fertilized before doing the procedure.

The doctor will slide a thin tube into your uterus and insert the sperm. According to Planned Parenthood, the process only takes between five and ten minutes and is generally painless. However, some women have experienced cramps afterward.

One of the benefits of IUI is that it generally costs less than the other procedures. It usually costs between three hundred and a thousand dollars, depending on how much the doctor's fees are. Some insurance plans will cover the procedure.

Surgery

Ray states that there are other surgical options that can help you get pregnant. Laparoscopic ovarian drilling is one such option. The doctor will use a laser to drill small holes in the ovaries. She says that this method is as effective as medications. It is sometimes used when medications have not worked.

There IS Hope

It is true that PCOS can make it harder to get pregnant. But, there are medications, supplements, and procedures that can help you become the great mother you are meant to be.

Dr. Emma Gray, who is a psychologist who specializes in people with fertility issues and suffers from PCOS herself, says that some people get pregnant as soon as they start trying, while other people have to try for a while. She says that it is not necessarily because one couple is more fertile than the other. It is a matter of luck and timing. More than eighty-five percent of couples conceive within the first year they start actively trying. The lesson here? Never give up.

Chapter Summary

● Because of insulin resistance and higher production levels of androgens, some women with PCOS may find it more difficult to become pregnant.

● Lifestyle changes, medications, and procedures can help you become fertile and pregnant.

Are you enjoying this book? Please consider leaving it a review!

In the next chapter, you will learn about how PCOS affects pregnancy.

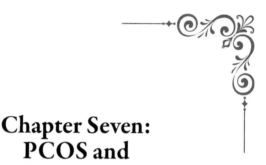

Chapter Seven:
PCOS and
Pregnancy

Regardless of what doctors predict and other people say, it is possible to get pregnant and deliver a healthy baby even if you have PCOS.

Remember Dr. Emma Gray from the end of the last chapter? She was diagnosed with PCOS at nineteen. She was told that it would be very difficult for her to have a child. At the time, she admits she didn't understand the gravity of what that really meant. For Dr. Gray, life went on. She decided to go to school and get a degree in psychology. Throughout her schooling, she found herself interested in working with people struggling mentally and emotionally because of fertility issues.

When Dr. Gray turned thirty-three, she began to understand what the idea of infertility really meant, emotionally speaking. She experienced, for herself, what her patients had been going through. She met and married a man, and together they wanted to have a family. She researched everything she could find on diet, exercise, supplements, and emotional well-being. She timed her ovulation periods.

After not having a period during her twenties and early thirties, she began to menstruate after making changes in her life. She soon became pregnant and gave birth to a healthy son. Soon, Dr. Gray and her husband decided they wanted another child, and she quickly became pregnant. Nine months later, she had another son. Two years later, she had a third son.

When she was forty-two, Dr. Gray and her husband decided they wanted a fourth child. It took her nine months to conceive. When she was ten weeks pregnant, she went in for a scan and found out that she had miscarried. Dr. Gray was devastated, but she and her husband tried to conceive again and six months later, she was pregnant. This time, she delivered her fourth son.

Dr. Gray's story is one of fear, determination, hope, happiness, devastation, and happiness again. Her story can be your story.

Polycystic ovary syndrome can create complications that you need to be aware of, so you can prepare for the arrival of a healthy baby. However, never doubt that a healthy baby can be a part of your future.

Miscarriages

Like everything else associated with PCOS, there is a lack of information regarding the association between PCOS and miscarriages. Some studies indicate that women who suffer from PCOS have an increased risk of having a miscarriage. However, Ray states that other studies attribute the miscarriages to being overweight or obese, fertility treatments, or increased age.

Dr. Gray cites a 2009 study conducted on one hundred forty-five women who suffered from PCOS. Seventy-nine of the women became pregnant and seventy-two of them delivered healthy babies. According to Dr. Gray this study demonstrates that the rate of miscarriages is not higher for women with PCOS. Every woman and every woman's body is different.

Originally, health experts thought that the miscarriage rate for women with PCOS was between thirty and fifty percent. Newer studies suggest that the rate might be even higher. Women who go through IVF or IUI tend to be twice as likely to have a miscarraige.

According to Nurse Galan, studies have shown that the risk factors for a miscarriage include insulin resistance, higher luteinizing hormone levels, elevated testosterone levels, obesity, infertility treatments, and genetics.

As with the other symptoms related to PCOS, there are steps that you can take to lessen your risk of suffering from a miscarriage.

1. Make lifestyle changes like exercising regularly and eating a healthy diet.
2. Galan states that Metformin not only helps improve your ability to get pregnant by lowering your insulin levels, it can also help you have a healthy pregnancy.
3. Bed rest or pelvic rest may also be advised by your doctor to help you have a successful pregnancy.

Sometimes miscarriages occur because there is a genetic abnormality. This is true for women who suffer from PCOS and for women who do not. This genetic abnormality means that the baby is not viable, and a miscarriage will occur.

Galan stresses that even if you have one miscarriage or multiple miscarriages, it is still possible to conceive and give birth to healthy babies.

Age is a mixed bag when it comes to becoming pregnant and delivering a healthy baby. As you get older, the symptoms of PCOS decrease, which makes it easier to become pregnant. However, age is also a factor in the risk of miscarriages. The older you are when you conceive, the higher the risk of having a miscarriage will be.

According to Dr. Gray, women with PCOS should start thinking of pregnancy as a twelve-month process instead of a nine-month process. First, it takes three months for eggs and sperm cells to mature. This means that your lifestyle choices including diet, exercise, smoking, medication, alcohol, and other choices you make four months before you conceive impact the quality of the egg and sperm. The greatest risk for the fetus to develop genetic abnormalities and birth defects exists when the fetus is between two and eight weeks. Therefore, fertility experts state that you should start planning your pregnancy at least three months before you begin trying to conceive.

Knowledge can be a powerful thing. The more information you have at your disposal, the easier it will be for you to take control of your experience. Despite her own struggles with pregnancy, Dr. Gray found the courage to keep going by learning more about her body: "My fertility journey has been full of surprises: the pain of miscarriage, as well as a healthy, naturally occurring pregnancy at 44 (the odds of which are low). Learning about my hormone levels, as well as keeping track of my cycle, made me feel empowered and gave me reason to keep trying."

Gestational Diabetes

Because they often have higher insulin levels, one of the issues faced by women with PCOS is gestational diabetes. There are other risk factors for gestational diabetes such as becoming pregnant when you are older than twenty-five, are overweight, have prediabetes, or have close relatives who have been diagnosed with type 2 diabetes.

Gestational diabetes can cause higher birth weight, respiratory problems at birth, low blood sugar, jaundice, and preterm birth. It can also make the birthing process more difficult for both the mother and the child.

In addition, gestational diabetes can cause the mother to develop type 2 diabetes later on.

Most of the time, women who develop gestational diabetes do not notice any of the symptoms. Galan states that rarely a woman might notice that she is experiencing excessive thirst and urination.

All women are tested for gestational diabetes when they are between twenty-four and twenty-eight weeks of pregnancy. Women with PCOS are often screened earlier in their pregnancy because of their increased risks.

According to a study conducted by the Endocrine Society, Metformin does not prevent gestational diabetes. Four hundred eighty-seven women participated in the study. Two hundred eleven of them received two thousand milligrams of Metformin each day. The other two hundred twenty-three received a placebo. According to the study, both groups had the same percentage of gestational diabetes.

Dr. Tone Loevvik, the doctor in charge of the study, said that while these results were disappointing, they reinforced what researchers had learned from previous studies.

The doctor may use one of two methods to screen for gestational diabetes. For both methods, you would drink a sugary liquid. If the doctor is screening using the glucose challenge, the doctor will draw your blood an hour after you have drunk the solution. You do not have to fast before doing this test. If the test results are not normal, then the doctor will perform the glucose challenge test. Some doctors do not do the glucose challenge at all and jump straight to the glucose tolerance test.

For the glucose tolerance test, you will need to fast prior to the test. Before drinking the sugary solution, the doctor will draw your blood. Then, the doctor will take your blood the one hour mark, the two hour mark, and the three hour mark after you drink the sugary liquid. If elevated glucose levels are found, then you will be diagnosed with gestational diabetes.

Once you are diagnosed, you will be asked to take your blood sugar levels a couple times a day. Galan states that you will likely need to check your levels when you wake up and after each meal.

Gestational diabetes is treated with lifestyle changes, such as light exercise and diet. You will need to eliminate processed and refined sugars, as well as fried or fatty foods. Your diet should mainly consist of fruits, vegetables, whole grains, and lean meat. The doctor will be able to recommend some light exercises you can do.

If the diet and exercise are not enough to treat the diabetes, the doctor will likely prescribe medication to control the blood sugar or insulin. Galan says that the doctor will tell you exactly what your treatment protocol should be. The doctor will also provide instructions about what your sugar levels should be at different points throughout the day. You will be provided with guidelines as to when you should call the doctor and when you should go to the hospital. It is very important that you follow your doctor's instructions.

Pregnancy Induced Hypertension and Preeclampsia

Both of these conditions affect women with and without PCOS. Because of the insulin resistance, women with PCOS tend to have higher blood pressure than other women. This increases your chance of developing one or both of these conditions during your pregnancy.

Pregnancy Induced Hypertension (PIH) refers to a condition where women develop high blood pressure after twenty weeks of pregnancy.

Preeclampsia is a gestational condition that may also appear during the second half of the pregnancy. In addition to high blood pressure, protein begins to appear in the urine. The protein in the urine causes you to swell. It is an indication that there is a problem with the kidneys.

If the preeclampsia is not treated, then it can develop into eclampsia. This can cause you to have seizures, become blind, or lapse into a coma. It can also result in your death or the death of your child. The good news is that this very rarely happens because doctors will monitor your health closely to make sure that you do not develop this health problem.

If you start experiencing swelling, have headaches, experience sudden weight gain, or have changes in your vision, you need to contact your doctor immediately. To check for PIH and preeclampsia, your doctor will check your blood pressure and take urine specimens every time you visit.

In the event that PIH or preeclampsia is diagnosed, you will be put on bed rest and monitored frequently. You will receive medication to lower your blood pressure. If your blood pressure does not decrease, the only cure is for the baby to be delivered. Your doctor will wait as long as possible before delivering the baby so the lungs have more time to develop.

Premature Birth

Women with PCOS are at a higher risk of delivering their babies prematurely, although Galan states that health experts are not entirely sure why this is the case. One of the reasons is that women with PCOS have a higher risk of PIH and preeclampsia. Galan states that another reason is that the babies tend to be bigger than normal for their gestational age.

However, a recent study of four hundred eighty-seven pregnant women who suffer from PCOS indicated that Metformin may once again be the answer. The women were from Norway, Sweden, and Iceland, and the average age was twenty-nine. The women were randomly assigned to take a placebo or two thousand milligrams of Metformin. The participants did not know which they received.

Researchers discovered that the combined rate of miscarrige in the second trimester and premature birth, where the women delivered at less than thirty-seven weeks, was almost halved for the women who took the Metformin. Researchers reported that only nine of the two hundred eleven women who took Metformin had either a premature birth or suffered a late-term miscarriage. These nine women represented five percent of the women who were taking the Metformin.

In contrast, ten percent, or twenty-three, of the two hundred twenty-three women who received the placebo, experienced either a late-term miscarriage or premature birth.

During the Pregnancy

There are several ways that you can take care of yourself during your pregnancy to ensure that you have a healthy pregnancy. One way is to monitor your diet. The PCOS Awareness Association states that you should work with a nutritionist who can help you develop a healthy diet. The diet will make sure that you and your baby get the right amount of nutrients and that you gain the right amount of weight during your pregnancy. You may be asked to restrict your carbohydrates during your pregnancy. The nutritionist may also recommend that you eat three small meals a day and have two to four healthy snacks in between.

Prenatal vitamins will be prescribed while you are pregnant. The doctor will work with you to determine which vitamins you will need. The PCOS Awareness Association states that the doctor will likely decrease your folic acids after the first trimester.

Physical activity is another important ingredient for a healthy pregnancy. Your doctor can help you find the right type of activity to take part in and determine how much of it you should do.

Delivery

Babies of women with PCOS tend to be large for their gestational age. For that reason, you may need to deliver through Cesarean section instead of delivering vaginally. Because this is a surgical procedure, you will need a longer time to recover. Although there is an increased risk to the mother and the baby, Cesarean births are not uncommon.

Breastfeeding

You are encouraged to breastfeed your baby. Not only are the nutrients in your milk good for the baby, the process creates a bond between you and your baby and it is also healthy for you. This is especially true if you are a diabetic.

1. Breastfeeding lowers your child's risk for childhood obesity. It also decreases the chances that your baby will develop type 2 diabetes later on in life.
2. If you suffer from gestational diabetes while you were pregnant, you are at an increased risk of developing type 2 diabetes later on. However, breastfeeding decreases the chances that you will develop type 2 diabetes.
3. Insulin and Metformin are safe when you are breastfeeding.
4. Breastfeeding helps you lose weight faster.

Have a Healthy, Safe Pregnancy and Delivery

Regardless of statistics and what doctors tell you, having a healthy pregnancy is possible. As Jen Bell states, women with PCOS tend to have the same number of children during their lifetimes, as do women without the syndrome. Other women, such as Dr. Emma Gray, Stephanie, and Amy, will testify to the fact that not only can you get pregnant, but you can have a healthy pregnancy and deliver happy, healthy babies.

Chapter Summary

- Many women with PCOS have multiple, healthy children.

- Women with PCOS may be more likely to have pregnancy complications. However, the doctors will be monitoring your pregnancy and will treat any issues.

- While late-term miscarriages and preterm births are more common for women with PCOS, studies show that Metformin can greatly decrease these risks.

- Breastfeeding is encouraged, even if you are diabetic.

In the next chapter, you will learn about microbiomes and how they can benefit you.

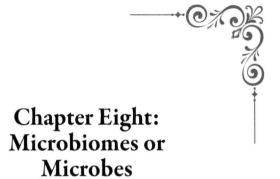

Chapter Eight:
Microbiomes or
Microbes

B acteria and viruses are not simply invisible threats that fly around outside of our bodies trying to make us sick. Fungi are not simply the mushrooms we put in our food or the toadstools that happy fairies dance around. They live, by the trillions, inside of our bodies. These invisible living organisms are known as microorganisms or microbes.

Bacteria, viruses, and fungi are often associated with illness and disease. However, specific types of these organisms are necessary for good health. Most of them live on your skin or in your large intestine. The microbes that live in your large intestine are referred to as the gut microbiome.

Dr. Ruairi Robertson provides this somewhat scary fact: "[T]here are more bacterial cells in your body than human cells. There are roughly 40 trillion bacterial cells in your body and only 30 trillion human cells. That means you are more bacteria than human."

There are more than one thousand species of bacteria that live in your gut microbiome alone. Most of them are essential for good health.

The microbes act as an additional organ in your body. Of this, Dr. Robertson says, "Altogether, these microbes may weigh as much as 2–5 pounds (1–2 kg), which is roughly the weight of your brain. Together, they function as an extra organ in your body and play a huge role in your health."

Studies show that you are exposed to microbes when you are still in the womb. As you grow, the number of microbes and microbe species expands. The higher your microbe diversity, the better your health will be.

Gut microbes are important for your health for a variety of reasons:

1. Gut microbes begin helping you at a very young age. They even help you digest the sugars in breast milk that are essential for growth.
2. Some of the bacteria in the microbes help digest fiber, which then produces short-chain fatty acids. This is especially important for women with PCOS because the fiber helps prevent weight gain, diabetes, and heart disease. Fiber also helps decrease your risk for cancer.
3. Although it does sound contradictory, the gut bacteria and other microorganisms in your body promote immunity. The gut microbiome communicates with your immune system, advising it on how to respond.
4. New research suggests that healthy gut microbiomes also affect the central nervous system, including the brain, which means that gut microbes are essential for a healthy brain.

Studies indicate that women with PCOS tend to have a smaller gut biome diversity than women who do not. Dr. Varykina Thackray states that this is likely because women with PCOS tend to have elevated testosterone levels. "Our study suggests testosterone and other androgen hormones may help shape the gut microbiome, and these changes may influence the development of PCOS and the impact it has on a woman's quality of life."

Weight

Weight is an important issue for women with PCOS. As discussed earlier, not all women who suffer from PCOS are overweight or obese, which is why this book does not focus on weight loss and I wrote an entirely separate book on that topic. However, PCOS can cause weight gain and make it more difficult to shed that weight. The gut microbiomes may be able to provide one solution for this problem.

Dr. Robertson notes that there are thousands of different types of bacteria in your gut, the majority of which are healthy. However, there are some unhealthy bacteria that gather there as well. If you get too many of those bad guys hanging out together in your gut, they can cause diseases and other health problems.

There are several studies that have investigated the microbiomes found in identical twins where one twin is obese and the other is not. The studies showed that the differences between the twins were the microbiomes.

Dr. Robertson cites a study in which the microbiomes from obese twins was transferred to mice. The result was the mice that had the unhealthy microbiomes gained a lot of weight and became obese. The obese mice were on the same diet as the lean mice. The weight gain was not attributed to the food they were eating or the amount of food they were eating. The unhealthy microbiomes in the gut was determined to be the cause.

Blood Sugar and Diabetes

One of the major issues surrounding PCOS is insulin resistance, which gut microbiomes may influence.

A recent study on thirty-three infants, who were genetically predisposed to develop type 1 diabetes, showed that the diversity levels of the gut microbiomes dropped significantly just before the onset of the disease. The study also found that the number of unhealthy gut microbiomes increased just before the onset of the diabetes. This is an indication that the diversity of gut microbiomes could affect whether you are diagnosed with type 2 diabetes.

Studies have also shown that gut microbes and the diversity of gut microbes can impact blood sugar levels. By promoting a large diversity of microbiomes in your system, you can reduce your blood sugar, which in turn, can reduce insulin levels. This may not only reduce your risk for type 2 diabetes, but it can also help slow or even reverse some of your symptoms for PCOS.

Mental Health

The gut is connected to the brain via millions of nerves, making microbes essential for positive mental health. Dr. Robertson explains that the reason why the gut microbiome can affect your mental health is because it controls the messages that are sent to your brain. Crystal Raypole, writing for Healthline, says that this connection is referred to by experts as the gut-brain axis, or the GBA.

Some of the bacteria species encourage your brain to produce neurotransmitters. Serotonin, the chemical that is responsible for many positive emotions, including feelings of happiness and well-being, is mostly produced in the gut. Therefore, in order for the serotonin to be produced, healthy bacteria have to be present.

Other transmitters that are produced by the microbiomes are those that regulate your appetite and your sleep habits.

Maintaining a healthy microbiome can help reduce inflammation in your body, which in turn, can help reduce symptoms associated with depression.

In addition, the healthy biomes improve your brain function and your reaction to stress.

According to Raypole, "It's unclear how probiotics carry out these functions, but a 2015 research review suggests the GBA may be the "missing link" in our understanding of depression and its causes."

There are several studies that indicate that people who suffer from mental and emotional disorders have different species of microbes that reside in their gut compared to people who do not suffer from psychological issues. With this in mind, Dr. Robertson suggests there is a correlation between healthy gut biomes and healthy mental health.

Some studies have shown that certain probiotics can improve the symptoms of depression and other mental and emotional health issues.

Raypole states that some experts have labeled this group of microbiomes as psychobiotics. One study that was conducted in 2017 discovered that taking a daily probiotic helped improve the symptoms associated with depression and anxiety.

Research indicates that probiotics work best when they are taken along with other treatments, which might include medication and therapy.

According to Raypole, "Existing research on probiotics for depression and other mental health issues is largely promising, but many of the existing studies are very small. This makes it hard to know just how effective probiotics are for depression."

One important area experts need to focus on during their research is the different types of microbiomes since different types of biomes seem to affect mental illnesses differently. While microbiome A might affect depression and anxiety, microbiome B might affect bipolar disorder.

Another important issue that will need further research is dosage. Some mental health disorders will need different doses of probiotics.

Raypole states that this can be a particularly difficult area to research because mental health issues affect people differently, just as microbiomes affect people differently. "A number of factors, including genetics, bacterial exposure, and life experiences, can affect the unique composition of your gut bacteria. This, in turn, may impact both the depression symptoms you experience, as well as which probiotics will work best for you."

Other Health Issues Related to Microbiomes
Gut Related Issues

There are several health issues that are affected by the gut microbiomes. They are related to different intestinal diseases, such as irritable bowel syndrome and inflammatory bowel disease.

Certain types of bacteria, such as those found in yogurt and other probiotics, can fill in the gaps that exist between intestinal cells. This helps prevent leaky gut syndrome. These healthy bacteria also prevent unhealthy bacteria from sticking to the intestinal walls.

Heart Disease and Related Issues

Because of increased insulin resistance, weight gain, and other factors, women with PCOS are more at risk for metabolic syndrome, which are a collection of issues that can relate to heart disease. However, according to Dr. Robertson, healthy gut microbiomes may be able to help you lower your chances of having to deal with heart issues along with everything else.

He states that a recent study of fifteen hundred people showed that microbiomes played an important role in increasing HDL, the good cholesterol, and triglycerides.

There are some bad bacteria that change the nutrients that are found in red meat and other foods into a chemical called TMAO that contributes to block arteries. Probiotics may help eliminate the bad bacteria and promote good heart health.

Probiotics

Probiotics can be used to help create healthy levels of gut microbiomes. They are live bacteria that "reseed" your gut with healthy bacteria. They can be used to control your weight, although many studies suggest that the effects of probiotics on weight loss is actually small.

Web MD says that probiotics can help with many other issues such as:

1. irritable bowel syndrome
2. inflammatory bowel disease

3. infectious diarrhea
4. diarrhea caused by antibiotics
5. certain skin ailments like eczema
6. urinary health issues
7. vaginal health issues
8. oral health
9. preventing colds and allergies

There are many types of probiotics, but there are two main groups. One group is Lactobacillus and is likely the most common kind of bacteria. These microscopic organisms are found in yogurt and other fermented foods. They can help out with a lot of issues, including lactose intolerance and diarrhea.

Bifidobacterium is the other main bacteria group and is found in dairy products. This bacteria is especially helpful in dealing with issues like irritable bowel syndrome.

Other Ways to Promote Healthy Gut Microbiomes

Dr. Robertson suggests several ways you can increase your healthy gut biomes.

1. You should eat a variety of foods. A diverse range of food can result in a diverse range of biomes.
    Legumes, fruits, and beans have a lot of fiber in them and promote healthy bacteria.
2. Fermented foods, such as yogurt, sauerkraut, and kefir, have healthy bacteria in them. The bacteria from these foods help decrease the unhealthy bacteria that cause diseases.
3. Limit the amount of artificial sweeteners that you consume. Although many people use artificial

sweeteners to reduce their blood sugar, they may actually increase blood sugar by causing unhealthy bacteria to grow in your gut.

4. Eating a lot of prebiotic foods can help stimulate the production of healthy gut bacteria and other microbiomes. These foods include bananas, asparagus, artichokes, apples, and oats.

5. Breastfeeding for at least six months is important because it helps develop healthy gut microbiomes in babies.

6. Whole grains are also an important part of your diet. They contain a lot of fiber and healthy carbohydrates that can be digested by the microbiomes. Whole grains can help prevent weight gain and reduce your risk for diabetes and cancer.

7. Vegetarian diets are also beneficial for healthy gut biomes. They reduce unhealthy gut bacteria, such as e.coli. Vegetarian diets also reduce inflammation and bad cholesterol levels.

8. Foods that are rich in polyphenols are also important. Polyphenols, which are plant compounds, are found in foods that we love, such as red wine and dark chocolate. They are also found in green tea and whole grains. The gut bacteria break down the polyphenols and use them to grow healthy bacteria.

9. Only take antibiotics when it is absolutely necessary. Antibiotics kill unhealthy bacteria, but they also kill healthy bacteria.

More Research Needed

According to Thackray, "Additional research is needed to determine whether specific gut bacterial species contribute to the development of PCOS and whether the microbiome offers potential pathways for treating the condition.

If testosterone drives the microbial composition of the gut, a compelling next step would be to determine if treatment of PCOS with testosterone blockers or oral contraceptives results in the recovery of the gut microbiome. It would also be important to figure out whether the gut microbiome of women diagnosed with PCOS using the criteria of polycystic ovaries and irregular or no menstrual periods is distinct from the gut microbiome of women diagnosed with the other subtypes of PCOS that require elevated testosterone."

The Ally Organ You Never Knew You Had

By increasing the number of healthy gut microorganisms that live inside of your body, you can control your weight gain, insulin levels, and decrease your chances of developing cancer and metabolic syndrome. You may also be able to control the depression and anxiety that often accompanies the PCOS. These trillions of tiny live microorganisms can make a huge difference in your life.

Chapter Summary

- You have trillions of tiny organisms inside of your body that influence different aspects of your health. This includes weight, insulin, heart health, and even mental health.

- Women with PCOS tend to have a smaller diversity of healthy microbiomes.

- There are ways to increase your healthy gut microbiomes and improve your overall health.

- Healthy gut microbiomes may result in relief and even reversal of some of your PCOS symptoms.

The next chapter will discuss the mindset for moving forward.

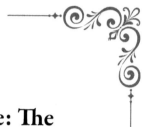

Chapter Nine: The Mindset for Moving Forward

Millions of women are diagnosed with PCOS each year. Many more do not even know they have it. Despite it being a health issue that affections a large part of the world's population and that it is considered to be the most significant cause of infertility, there is still relatively little known about this disease.

Speak Up for Yourself if You Have Symptoms

If you are experiencing any of the symptoms of PCOS, get checked out. If the first doctor dismisses your thoughts and fears, then go to another. Keep going to different doctors until you find someone who will listen to you.

One woman told *Clue* that she had gone to see a regular doctor several times about her irregular period. She was told that her period would straighten itself out when she was older. It never did. She went to a specialist and demanded more testing. The specialist obliged, and she was finally able to get help. The woman said that she wishes she had gone to a specialist earlier instead of suffering through the symptoms for so long. She urged anyone suffering to seek out treatment saying, "If you think you might have PCOS: speak up, there's an answer. You can get help, get more testing done."

If you are overweight or obese, doctors may ignore your complaints. Stay strong, and be prepared to advocate for yourself because regardless of how much you weigh, your concerns and struggles are still valid.

One woman told *Clue* that she dealt with the symptoms of PCOS for fifteen years before she could find a doctor that would help her. She had excessive hair growth, irregular periods, acne, hair loss, and difficulty losing weight. Though one doctor admitted that she likely did have PCOS, the only advice/treatment she received was an instruction to lose weight. Four more doctors told her exactly the same thing: lose weight. Because her weight was all they would focus on, she felt dismissed because of her size and it kept her from speaking up and getting treatment sooner. She eventually found a specialist who took her seriously and offered her the treatment she needed. She encourages others to keep fighting for themselves saying, "My advice? Keep pushing for a diagnosis. Sometimes test results aren't definitive but you know if something isn't right. If you don't get help and advice, exercise your right to see a different doctor until you get the help you deserve."

PCOS Is Not the Same for Everyone

Polycystic ovary syndrome does not affect every woman the same. Some women experience all the symptoms, while others may not suffer any at all. Some women have cysts and some do not.

One woman from France told *Clue* that though she was diagnosed with PCOS, since she did not suffer from any outward symptoms, they did not do regular checkups. As a result, she was not informed or prepared for issues like infertility, painful cysts, or painful ovulation.

Part of the reason that there is very little known about PCOS is because there are so many different parts to it. Unlike other diseases, such as cancer, where there is a specific target that can be identified and dealt with, PCOS is a multi-branched tree.

Another reason is that the disease affects everyone differently. One woman could have ovarian cysts, while another does not. One woman could be overweight, another could be obese, while a third is lean. There seems to be little consistency between the disease and its effects.

Yet another barrier is the name. Health experts that specialize in PCOS are advocating that the name be changed to better reflect what it actually is: An endocrine issue. The syndrome seems to be more about insulin resistance and the effects of higher insulin levels, which indirectly, includes multiple cysts on and in the ovaries.

Take Charge of Your Symptoms, Your Syndrome, Your Body, and Your Life

Many women with PCOS have struggled with the disease for years. Many have dealt with doctors who have not taken their condition seriously. Even doctors who do take the disease seriously are often ignorant or misinformed.

You can take control of your symptoms. You can even reverse some of your symptoms. However, it is extremely important that YOU CONSULT A DOCTOR BEFORE TAKING SUPPLEMENTS, PROBIOTICS, OR CHANGING YOUR DIET. Every woman is different. Every woman presents different symptoms and different side effects. Put your safety first and make sure your have medical support before adopting any drastic changes.

Many women are told that it would be impossible or nearly impossible to become pregnant, especially without fertility treatments. Yet many women, such as Dr. Gray, Stephanie, and Amy, have not only conceived but delivered healthy babies.

There are many other issues, including acne, excessive hair growth, thinning hair, and male pattern baldness, that seem to add insult to injury. While there are cosmetic ways to treat many of these issues, some women, like model Hernaam Kaur, have decided to simply live with them and love themselves for who they are. There is no "right" answer except following your instincts and doing what feels "right" for you.

For most women, lifestyle changes seem to help a lot. Exercising daily for thirty to sixty minutes not only helps with weight loss and decreases your insulin levels, but it also helps improve mental health. Eating a good, healthy diet is also important and can even include delicious foods and drinks like dark chocolate and red wine.

It is important to remember that PCOS is not who you are. It is a syndrome you have. You are so much more than a syndrome. You are an amazing, strong, beautiful woman who overcomes the struggle that life throws at her, one step at a time. You are on a journey that will lead you to a fulfilling life and happiness. The secret to a successful journey is to love yourself despite the struggles that PCOS throws in your path.

It is extremely important that you love yourself. This is not always an easy task, but it is an important one. You may be tired, cranky, and sore. You might have extra hair or thinning hair with a bad case of acne. This is not who you are. It is a symptom of a syndrome you have. It does not define you, and it does not take away from your beauty. You might not feel lovable. This is okay. Love yourself anyway.

Loving yourself means that you forgive yourself. Even if last night you were hanging out with friends, ate a bunch of tacos or pizza and drank too much soda, completely wrecking your diet, that is okay. Sometimes, we fall off the wagon. Dust yourself off and get back up on it. You only fail when you do not try.

Loving yourself also means being your own advocate. Talk with your doctor to determine the best treatments for you. If you believe that your doctor is not helping you or giving you the answers you seek, then do not hesitate to seek a second opinion, or even a third or fourth opinion.

Taking care of your mental and emotional health is another aspect of loving yourself. It is easy to get overwhelmed when trying to deal with the symptoms of PCOS on top of everyday life. This makes it too easy to ignore the depression or anxiety until it reaches a point that it takes over your life. Evaluate your mental state every so often, and do not be afraid to reach out to others if you need to.

We leave off with one final inspiring story of a woman who conquered her PCOS:

Christina Espinoza, a mother of two children, took charge of her life and decreased some of the symptoms associated with her PCOS. Christina took part in a study conducted by UC Davis Health where she was asked to eat a certain number of walnuts every day. But she didn't stop at just eating walnuts. Christina also made healthy lifestyle changes in an effort to improve her life. Exercising five to seven days per week helped her go down in clothing sizes from a thirteen to an eight. She experienced an increase energy levels and her periods are now normal. Before she would spend at least thirty minutes every day plucking her facial hair. Now, she only spends between fifteen and twenty minutes plucking. She loves the fact that her facial hair does not grow as much anymore. Perhaps the change she is happiest with is that she's now decreased her risks of heart attack, stroke, and type 2 diabetes. Christina contends that the lifestyle changes she made, in addition to adding walnuts to her diet, had a tremendous impact on her PCOS and its symptoms.

More health experts are aware of PCOS and they are searching for answers. In the meantime, take comfort in knowing you are not alone. Like Christina, Dr. Gray, Stephanie, Amy, and millions of other women, you can change your life for the better and survive PCOS.

Chapter Summary

- Make sure you check with a doctor before you make any lifestyle changes or take supplements.

- There is hope for the reversal of some, if not all, symptoms of PCOS.

- Do not be afraid to speak up for yourself.

- You are not alone.

I hope you have enjoyed the content in this book and, most importantly, learned something that you can apply in your effort to live a better life with PCOS. If you are also interested in learning what dieting methods are best for those with PCOS, please check out the companion book, THE PCOS DIET, also written by me.

If you enjoyed this book, **please consider leaving a review!** This is a huge help for me and helps me to put out more content like this. Thanks again, and good luck on your journey ahead.

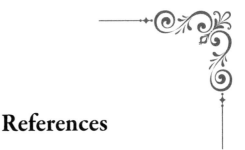

References

Bell, J. (September 10, 2018). Managing PCOS symptoms: Experiences and advice. Retrieved from https://helloclue.com/articles/cycle-a-z/managing-pcos-symptoms-experiences-and-advice

Bell, J. (November 6, 2018). PCOS: Myths and facts about symptoms, diagnosis, and treatments. Retrieved from https://helloclue.com/articles/cycle-a-z/what-you-may-not-know-about-pcos-questions-and-misconceptions.

Briden, L. M.D. (September 3, 2018). PCOS and insulin resistance—testing and treatment. Retrieved from https://helloclue.com/articles/cycle-a-z/the-link-be-tween-pcos-and-insulin-resistance

Brown, M.J. Ph.D. (December 22, 2016). Advanced glyca-tion end products (AGEs). Retrieved from https://www.healthline.com/nutrition/advanced-glycation-end-products.

CCRM Fertility. (2019). PCOS and infertility. Retrieved from https://www.ccrmivf.com/pcos-infertility/.

Center for Young Women's Health. (February 25, 2014).
PCOS: Insulin and Metformin.

Retrieved from https://youngwomenshealth.org/2014/
02/25/metformin/.

Cherney, K. (November 2, 2018). Polycystic ovary syndrome (PCOS) and acne: Connection,

treatment, and more. Retrieved from https://www.health-
line.com/health/pcos-acne.

Clark, M. (May 30, 2018). 5 women with PCOS explain
why they choose to celebrate their facial

hair. Retrieved from
https://www.allure.com/story/women-with-pcos-facial-
hair-beard-interviews.

Endocrine Society. (March 20, 2018). Metformin lowers
risk of late miscarriage and preterm

births in women with PCOS. Retrieved from
https://www.endocrine.org/news-room/2018/met-
formin-lowers-risk-of-late-miscarriage-pret
erm-birth-in-pregnant-women-with-pcos.

Galan, N. (April 22, 2019). Androgenic alopecia in women
who have PCOS. Retrieved from
https://www.verywellhealth.com/androgenic-alope-
cia-2616683.

Galan, N. (April 28, 2019). Are there painless forms of hair
removal. Retrieved from
https://www.verywellhealth.com/are-there-painless-
forms-of-hair-removal-2616681.

Galan, N. (April 24, 2019). Dealing with the side effects of
waxing. Retrieved from

https://www.verywellhealth.com/dealing-with-the-side-effects-of-waxing-2616682.

Galan, N. (April 24, 2019). Gestational diabetes. Retrieved from
https://www.verywellfamily.com/what-is-gestational-diabetes-2616348.

Galan, N. (May 3, 2019). Permanent hair removal for women with PCOS. Retrieved from
https://www.verywellhealth.com/what-you-need-to-know-before-having-electrolysis-26166
89.

Galan, N. (April 27, 2019). Pregnancy complications associated with PCOS. Retrieved from
https://www.verywellhealth.com/potential-pregnancy-complications-with-pcos-2616640.

Galan, N. (July 7, 2019). Risk factors relating to PCOS and miscarriages. Retrieved from
https://www.verywellhealth.com/pcos-miscarriage-rate-what-are-the-risks-factors-2616653.

Gray, E. (March 21, 2019). My fertility story: PCOS, pregnancy, and surprise. Retrieved from
https://modernfertility.com/blog/dr-emma-gray/.

Greenlaw, E. (2019). How antidepressants and depression medication can affect your life.
Retrieved from https://www.webmd.com/depression/features/antidepressant-effects#1.

Harrar, S. (2019). Polycystic ovary syndrome (PCOS): How is it diagnosed? Retrieved from https://www.endocrineweb.com/conditions/poly-cystic-ovary-syndrome-pcos/polycystic-ovary-syn-drome-pcos-how-it-diagnosed.

Harrar, S. (2019). What causes PCOS? And how will it affect my body? Retrieved from

https://www.endocrineweb.com/conditions/poly-cystic-ovary-syndrome-pcos/what-causes-pcos-how-will-it-affect-body.

Harvard Health. (April 30, 2018). Exercise is an all-natural treatment to fight depression.
Retrieved from

https://www.health.harvard.edu/mind-and-mood/exercise-is-an-all-natural-treatment-to-fight-depres-sion.

Harvard Health. (August 2018). How meditation helps with depression. Retrieved from
https://www.health.harvard.edu/mind-and-mood/how-meditation-helps-with-depression.

Healthline. (2019). Top 15 calcium-rich foods (Many are non-dairy). Retrieved from
https://www.healthline.com/nutrition/15-calcium-rich-foods.

Healthline. (2019). Yoga and depression: How does it work? Retrieved from
https://www.healthline.com/health/depression/yoga-therapy.

Jennings, K. (August 28, 2018). 16 simple ways to relieve stress and anxiety. Retrieved from
https://www.healthline.com/nutrition/16-ways-relieve-stress-anxiety.

Khaleeli, H. (September 13, 2016). The lady with a beard: "If you've got it, rock it!". Retrieved
from
https://www.theguardian.com/fashion/2016/sep/13/lady-with-a-beard-if-youve-got-it-rock-it
-guinness-world-records

Klein, A. (May 14, 2018). Cause of polycystic ovarian syndrome discovered at last. *New*

Scientist. Retrieved   from   https://www.newscientist.com/article/2168705-cause-of-polycystic-ovary-syndrome-discovered-at-last/.

Konstantinvosky, M. (January 14, 2019). 6 natural treatments for PCOS. Retrieved from
https://www.onemedical.com/blog/get-well/pcos-treatment.

Lusinski, N. (October 5, 2018). The most ridiculous things women with PCOS are told by their
doctors. Retrieved from
https://www.bustle.com/p/the-most-ridiculous-things-women-with-pcos-were-told-by-their-
doctors-12165657.

Mayo Clinic. (2019). Cognitive behavioral therapy. Retrieved from https://www.mayoclinic.org/tests-procedures/cognitive-behavioral-therapy/about/pac-2038610.

Mayo Clinic. (2019). Depression and anxiety: Exercise eases symptoms. Retrieved from
https://www.mayoclinic.org/diseases-conditions/depression/in-depth/depression-and-exercis
e/art-20046495

Mayo Clinic. (2019). Polycystic ovary syndrome (PCOS). Retrieved from

https://www.mayoclinic.org/diseases-conditions/pcos/diagnosis-treatment/drc-20353443.

Migala, J. (May 31, 2018). What are the symptoms of PCOS, and how is the health condition
diagnosed? Retrieved from https://www.everydayhealth.com/pcos/symptoms-diagnosis/.

Mindful Staff. (January 31, 2019). How to meditate. Retrieved from
https://www.mindful.org/how-to-meditate/.

News Wise. (January 23, 2018). Women with polycystic ovaries syndrome have less bacterial
diversity in gut. Retrieved from
https://www.newswise.com/articles/women-with-polycystic-ovary-syndrome-have-less-bact
erial-diversity-in-gut.

Paddock, C. Ph.D. (July 3, 2017). How to give up smoking: 10 tips. Retrieved from
https://www.medicalnewstoday.com/articles/241302.php.

PCOS Awareness Association. (2019). Pcos pregnancy and delivery complications. Retrieved
    from https://www.pcosaa.org/pcos-pregnancy-and-delivery-complications.

Planned Parenthood. (2019). What is in-vitro fertilization (IVF)? Retrieved from
    https://www.plannedparenthood.org/learn/pregnancy/fertility-treatments/what-ivf.

Planned Parenthood. (2019). What is intrauterine Insemination (IUI)? Retrieved from
    https://www.plannedparenthood.org/learn/pregnancy/fertility-treatments/what-iui.

Powell, R. (April 27, 2018). Polycystic ovary syndrome: Women tell their stories of their
    debilitating condition. Retrieved from
    https://www.abc.net.au/news/2018-04-28/polycystic-ovary-syndrome-women-on-life-with-pcos/9607494.

Ray, L. (October 10, 2018). Depression, anxiety, and PCOS. Retrieved from
    https://helloclue.com/articles/cycle-a-z/depression-anxiety-and-pcos.

Ray, L. (August 23, 2018). PCOS and pregnancy. Retrieved from
    https://helloclue.com/articles/cycle-a-z/pcos-and-pregnancy.

Rapole, C. (March 21, 2019). Can probiotics help with depression? Retrieved from
    https://www.healthline.com/health/probiotics-depression.

Reese, A. (November 6, 2017). Mental health screening should accompany PCOS diagnosis.

Retrieved from https://www.healio.com/en-docrinology/reproduction-androgen-disorders/news/on-line/%7bf0f9e864-b429-4714-8a51-16c565aa07df%7d/mental-health-screening-should-accompany-pcos-diagnosis.

Rewire Me. (2019). 5 breathing exercises to reduce anxiety and depression. Retrieved from https://www.rewireme.com/mindfulness-happiness/5-breathing-exercises-reduce-anxiety-depression/.

Robertson, R. (July 27, 2017). Why the gut microbiome is crucial for your health. Retrieved from https://www.healthline.com/nutrition/gut-microbiome-and-health.

Ruled.Me. (2019). HOw to reverse polycystic ovary syndrome. Retrieved from https://www.ruled.me/reverse-polycystic-ovary-syndrome-pcos-naturally/.

Santos-Longhurst, A. (March 8, 2019). How to manage PCOS-related hair loss. Retrieved from https://www.healthline.com/health/pcos-hair-loss-2.

Sharpe, A. (August 15, 2018). The foods that balance out (or mess with) your hormones. Retrieved from https://greatist.com/eat/foods-for-hormonal-imbalance#1.

Spritzler, F. (August 22, 2019). 10 magnesium-rich foods that are super healthy. Retrieved from https://www.healthline.com/nutrition/10-foods-high-in-magnesium

Teede, H. (July 27, 2018). New international PCOS guideline aims to streamline care. Retrieved

fromhttps://www.healio.com/endocrinology/re-production-androgen-disorders/news/in-the-jour-nals/%7bd46d7f0c-bd76-4df2-926b-31ae5130f570%7d/new-interna-tional-pcos-guideline-aims-to-streamline-care.

UC Davis researchers look to new PCOS treatments. (2019). Retrieved from https://health.ucdavis.edu/welcome/features/20070919_pcos/.

Vann, M. (November 13, 2017). How to maintain a healthy body image. Retrieved from https://www.everydayhealth.com/eating-disorders/how-to-have-a-healthy-body-image.aspx.

Villines, Z. (November 17, 2017). Best birth control pills for PCOS. Retrieved from https://www.medicalnewstoday.com/articles/320055.php.

Watson, K. (April 6, 2018). Natural treatment PCOS: 30 natural ways to help treat polycystic ovary syndrome. Retrieved from https://docs.google.com/document/d/1LYTh1TPIXjsG-zlvrr6N3Pd8lKTqml3FihvG4y-j0fE/

edit.

Watson, S. (November 1, 2018). Polycystic ovarian syndrome (PCOS): Symptoms, causes, and
treatment. Retrieved from https://www.healthline.com/health/polycystic-ovary-disease.

WebMD. (2019). Chromium supplement: Health benefits and risks. Retrieved from
https://www.webmd.com/diet/supplement-guide-chromium#1.

WebMD. (2019). Depression and diet. Retrieved from
https://www.webmd.com/depression/guide/diet-recovery#1.

WebMD. (2019). Sleep and depression. Retrieved from
https://www.webmd.com/depression/guide/depression-sleep-disorder#1.

WebMD. (2019). What are probiotics? Retrieved from
https://www.webmd.com/digestive-disorders/what-are-probiotics#1.

West, H. (April 19, 2018). The 10 best foods that are high in zinc. Retrieved from
https://www.healthline.com/nutrition/best-foods-high-in-zinc.

What is PCOS? (2019). Retrieved from
https://www.girlshealth.gov/body/reproductive/pcos.html.

Zhang, B., Shen, S., & Zhu, D. (July 2018). Gut Microbiota as a potential target for treatment of
polycystic ovary syndrome. Retrieved from
https://diabetes.diabetesjournals.org/content/67/Supplement_1/2454-PUB.

CPSIA information can be obtained
at www.ICGtesting.com
Printed in the USA
LVHW081158261221
707160LV00021B/739

9 781951 745011